CEREBRAL PALSY IN CHILDHOOD

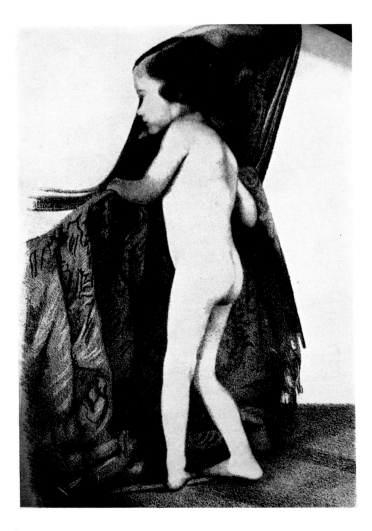

Drawing of a case of spasticity from Little's original article in the
Transactions of the Obstetrical Society, London, 1862, **3**, 293.

CEREBRAL PALSY IN CHILDHOOD

(THE AETIOLOGY AND CLINICAL ASSESSMENT
WITH PARTICULAR REFERENCE TO THE FINDINGS
IN BRISTOL)

BY

GRACE E. WOODS, M.D., D.P.H., D.C.H.
Deputy Medical Superintendent of Hortham Hospital

WITH A FOREWORD BY

PETER HENDERSON, M.D., D.P.H.
Principal Medical Officer, Ministry of Education

BRISTOL: JOHN WRIGHT & SONS LTD.

1957

PRINTED IN GREAT BRITAIN BY
JOHN WRIGHT & SONS LTD.
AT THE STONEBRIDGE PRESS,
BRISTOL

PREFACE

DURING the past few years many articles have appeared in medical journals about various aspects of infantile cerebral palsy. From these articles, it is obvious that this disease is not a single entity, but a collection of clinical conditions which have in common two factors only. Firstly, there is a disease of the brain. Secondly, there is in consequence a defect of movement. This book is an attempt to analyse the aetiology of all the varying cerebral palsies in childhood, which may be antenatal, natal, or postnatal in origin, and to give at the same time a description of the child's other defects, such as deafness or sensory loss, and thus a clinical assessment of the whole child. It is an elaboration of an M.D. Thesis presented to the University of Bristol in March, 1956.

The survey on which these findings are based has been carried out during the last five years in Bristol, and has been assisted by research grants from the United Bristol Hospitals and the National Spastics Society. I would like to express my gratitude to these bodies.

I have also received invaluable assistance from many sources. I have to acknowledge the help and advice given me by Professor A. V. Neale, under whose direction the work has been carried out. I also wish to thank Dr. B. D. Corner and Dr. J. Apley for allowing me to see their cases. Dr. A. L. Smallwood has been of particular assistance in providing details of all the cerebral palsied children known to the Bristol Education Authority. Many cases have been referred by the Somerset Education Authority.

Dr. R. M. Norman has frequently given invaluable advice in discussing the likely pathology of these cases. Dr. R. Walker obtained figures of familial incidence of epilepsy. The electro-encephalographic records have been taken by the staff of the Burden Neurological Institute under the direction of Professor F. L. Golla. Many clinical problems have been discussed with Dr. P. Polani, and problems of deafness with Dr. L. Fisch.

Mr. R. V. Saunders has carried out all the intelligence testing, and has made observations of the child's specific learning difficulties. Miss E. H. L. Duncan has checked the numerical findings and given statistical advice.

Many interesting and exact observations on these children have been made by the various physiotherapists, speech therapists, and occupational therapists, and have been particularly useful. I would especially wish to thank Miss M. Ram and the staff of Claremont School for Spastics, Bristol, for their interest and co-operation.

The photographs were taken by Mr. F. A. Godman and the staff of the Medical Photography Department of the University of Bristol. Miss H. Perren has kindly carried out a large part of the secretarial work.

Finally, I must show my appreciation of the parents who are anxious to further the knowledge of their children's handicap, and have co-operated fully in obtaining records of the children.

Bristol,   G. E. W.
   November, 1957.

CONTENTS

FOREWORD

By Peter Henderson, M.D., D.P.H.

Principal Medical Officer, Ministry of Education

One hundred years ago, Dr. William John Little, a physician at the London Hospital, gave, for the first time, a clear clinical description of cerebral palsy and noted its relationship to prematurity, difficult labour, and asphyxia neonatorum. In the years that have since passed, the infant death-rate has been substantially reduced, the control of some of the diseases that used to cripple many children has tightened, and medical and maternal care have greatly improved. Children born maimed and who once would have died in infancy now survive, and fewer of those born healthy are now deformed by disease in later childhood. The result has been that cerebral palsy now stands high, if not chief, among the conditions causing physical handicap in children. It was found in a survey in Bristol, which is the subject of this book, that the number of cerebral palsied children who reached the age of 5 years was 1·9 per 1000 live births. In recent years cerebral palsy in children has been studied by an increasing number of doctors and educationists and there have been many papers (some would say too many) and a number of books on the subject.

The particular merit of this book by Dr. Grace Woods is that it gives the findings of a team of workers at the Bristol Children's Hospital, under the combined direction of the Professor of Child Health at Bristol University and the Chief School Physician of the Bristol School Health Service, on a group of 301 children. The team included, in addition to Dr. Woods, a school doctor, the chief educational psychologist of the Bristol Child Guidance Clinic, and a health visitor ; the headmistress of the Bristol day special school for children with cerebral palsy was closely associated with it. The children attended the follow-up clinic frequently and those who were at the special school were under close daily observation : some of the children were known to Dr. Woods for fourteen years.

The investigation, management, and education of children with cerebral palsy require the close co-operation of doctor, therapist, health visitor, educationist, and parent. Although this book is concerned mainly with the causation and the clinical description of the many manifestations of cerebral palsy, it sets an admirable example of co-operation between doctor, nurse, psychologist, and teacher.

This is a first-rate clinical study, undertaken with insight and patience. The different types of defect are described according to the upset of movement pattern. It is stressed that spasticity is not static and may be present in one group of muscles and then in another, depending on the posture and movement of the child : " The cortex knows nothing of muscles, it knows only movements," wrote Hughlings Jackson and this is aptly quoted by Dr. Woods.

It has long been known that deafness is more prevalent among children with cerebral palsy than among the normal child population ; 20 of the 301 children in this study were found to have defective hearing, and of the 32 athetoids 10 were affected. The hearing defect was considered to be of two distinct types : high-frequency deafness and ' auditory agnosia '. It is, however, often difficult to test the hearing of children who are also severely disabled by cerebral palsy and the results of hearing tests have to be interpreted with caution. It may well be that with more experience, and improved testing technique, a diagnosis of ' auditory agnosia ' will be made less often in future. The effect of marked hearing loss on the educational progress of a child who is also heavily handicapped by cerebral palsy has not yet been fully assessed. It can be investigated thoroughly only by persons skilled and experienced in the special methods used in the teaching of deaf children, and of children with severe cerebral palsy.

In addition to deafness, poor intelligence, and physical infirmity affecting adversely the education of cerebral palsied children, a number also appear to have specific perceptual difficulties that impede the process of learning : some, for example, may not be able to tell right from left, or may have no idea of numbers, or are unable to distinguish between different shapes. There is evidence that these difficulties may arise from damage to the parietal lobes. Dr. Woods is convinced that it is as necessary to deal with these perceptual difficulties as it is to treat the defect of movement. She makes a strong plea for early diagnosis so that treatment can be begun early and the specific learning difficulties tackled in the pre-reading stage " before serious school work begins ".

This book does not discuss methods, or results, of treatment : that is not its purpose. It is, however, concerned with the causes of cerebral palsy. Since many severely affected children, after long years of expensive treatment and education, remain permanently incapacitated at the end of their school days it is of first importance that the causation of the condition should be investigated in the hope that measures can be devised to prevent its onset. Less than half the total number of children who were the subject of this study were born after a normal full-time birth following a normal pregnancy, yet there was little evidence of unskilled midwifery. It seems, therefore, that with present knowledge little further preventive action can be taken. The need for research is pressing since many children are involved and a substantial number, despite early diagnosis and skilled management, remain almost completely dependent on others for the rest of their days.

Much can happen to the developing baby during its nine months of intra-uterine life and there are likely to be many factors that may affect it adversely : their elucidation is one of the toughest tasks in medical research. The case histories of the 301 children investigated by Dr. Woods and her colleagues are recorded in detail and merit close study.

Dr. Woods has written a book that is notable for its wealth of clinical descriptions, revealing case histories, and for a wide review of the writings of others. It is a record of long and painstaking observation that challenges thought. No one, be he doctor, therapist, or teacher, who works with cerebral palsied children should miss reading it.

London,
   October, 1957.

ABBREVIATIONS

A.E.G.	-	-	Air-encephalogram
A.P.H.	-	-	Antepartum hæmorrhage
E.E.G.	-	-	Electro-encephalogram
E.S.N.	-	-	Educationally subnormal
E.T.A.	-	-	Elongation of tendo achillis
I.Q.	-	-	Intelligence Quotient
O.S.	-	-	Ordinary School
P.H.S.	-	-	Physically Handicapped School
Oc.C.	-	-	Occupational Centre
b. -	-	-	Born
B.B.A.	-	-	Born before arrival of doctor or midwife

PLATE V

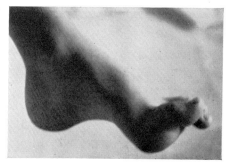

Fig. 11.—The foot in a case of left hemiplegia following vaccination. Loss of sense of position in toes has caused abrasion of his toe in his boot. There is marked spastic pes cavus.

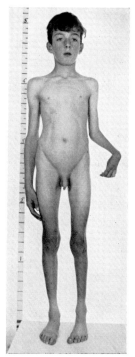

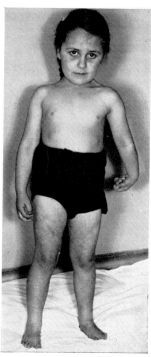

Fig. 12.—A case of left hemiplegia, with mental retardation, following empyema. A.E.G. showed bilateral lesion.

Fig. 13.—A case of hemi-athetosis following tuberculous meningitis. Possibly loss of body-image.

CEREBRAL PALSY IN CHILDHOOD

CHAPTER I

INTRODUCTORY

THE subject-matter of this book is based on the findings of cases referred to a Cerebral Palsy Assessment Clinic at the Bristol Royal Hospital for Sick Children. This clinic was run under the combined direction of Professor A. V. Neale, Professor of Child Health in the University of Bristol, and Dr. A. L. Smallwood, Chief School Physician, Bristol Health Services.

The prior purpose of the clinic was to assess the children for education and to place them in the most suitable school or occupation centre. It is likely that all cases between the ages of 5 and 17 years in the Administrative County of Bristol have been seen. Therefore the numbers are an accurate estimate of the proportion of cases of varying aetiology and movement defect in Bristol and possibly representative of the total population. The survey also includes some children under 5 years of age and many from outside the city boundary.

Cerebral palsy in childhood is the result of infantile cerebral palsy. It is, therefore, first necessary to define precisely what is meant by ' infantile cerebral palsy '. Courville (1950) defines it as " a clinical state resulting from some physical insult to the motor system of the developing or immature brain ". Perlstein (1949 b) says : " Cerebral palsy is a condition characterized by paralysis, weakness, inco-ordination or any other aberration of motor function due to pathology in the motor control centres of the brain". Thus the term 'infantile cerebral palsy' can be widely used to include all cases where there is an upset of the normal pattern of movement due to a cerebral cause. The cause may be an antenatal, natal, or post-natal damage or disease of the brain, and, using the term more widely than Courville, includes cases with a familial inheritance like hereditary spastic paraplegia. This wider definition will also include a number of cases which in the past have been crudely described as mentally defective. In many cases of mental deficiency there is a generalized rigidity, either mild or severe, which upsets normal movement. As will be shown later, some of these cases have a history of antenatal abnor-mality or obstetrical difficulty suggesting brain damage, and they can justifiably be included under the heading of cerebral palsy.

The term ' infantile cerebral palsy ' includes a wide variety of clinical conditions, and, as Phelps (1949) states, " Cerebral palsy differs from other handicapping conditions because it includes all functions of the brain. It does not represent only a motor handicap, but because of its origin in the brain may include mental and sensory deviations as well." Other cerebral functions such as sight, hearing, perception, understanding, feeling may also be defective to a different degree in each case, and because of the widespread or particular damage, no two cases are exactly alike.

It is customary when describing cerebral palsy cases to place them under definite headings such as (a) paraplegia ; (b) mono-plegia ; (c) hemiplegia ; (d) quadriplegia ; (e) athetosis ; (f) ataxia ; (g) rigidity. These terms describe only the upset in movement pattern, and under each heading are cases of different clinical conditions. In fact a case in one group may more closely resemble a case in another group than in its own. It is not always easy to be certain into which group a case should be put ; for example, a severe tension athetoid may at a single examination appear to be a case of spastic quadriplegia. As these cases can only be assessed by a personal appreciation of the movement upset and not, as will be shown later, by set clinical signs, there may be human errors of judgement in placing a case in one group rather than the other. These clinical subdivisions are artificial, and have been formed because the emphasis in cerebral palsy is on the movement upset.

After giving figures of comparative incidence the cases are discussed in chapters under the seven headings given above.

As they represent widely differing clinical conditions, overall statistics of the whole number can be very misleading, i.e., one cannot get a true picture of the significance of obstetric factors if one includes cases which appeared to originate after birth. On the other hand, if cases are analysed in groups which appear to represent one clinical condition, the numbers may be too small for statistical appraisal. The method of statistical analysis has been used guardedly and in many cases only statistical ' hunches ' can be made.

In each chapter a bald numerical statement is made of the findings, and then an attempt is made to show how the cases may be grouped under definite aetiological or clinical headings. As very few cases similar to the ones we are seeing have ever come to post-mortem, much of this work must remain conjectural, and striking similarities may even be coincidences.

The numerical findings of each movement-defect group are then analysed to show the significance of varying factors in the birth process in the causation of cerebral palsy.

Following this, there are four chapters elucidating the other neurological signs and symptoms found in these cases. As already mentioned, the emphasis in cerebral palsy is on defects of movement, but because the condition is due to brain pathology there may be a wide variety of other defects, often of more importance to the child and his future welfare than the movement handicap alone. The varieties of visual defects, speech and hearing defects, loss of sensory discrimination, and epileptiform disturbances are discussed separately.

In a final chapter an attempt is made to show that because of the widespread brain damage there is a disorientation of the child's whole personality which may involve a general lowering of intelligence, behaviour problems, and particular difficulties in perception and conception which affect the child's ability to master the tasks of education.

CHAPTER II

HISTORY AND LITERATURE

No survey of the literature on cerebral palsy can be begun without mentioning the work of Little. His practice as an orthopædic surgeon brought him into contact with cases of severe deformity following untreated cerebral palsy and he gives an account of these cases in his book *On Deformities* published in 1853. Of 7533 patients treated at the Orthopædic Institute, Bloomsbury Square, London, he considered that the deformities in 138 were due to nervous affection or paralysis, and although he suggested various causes for the condition, such as diarrhœa and internal upsets, he noted that a large proportion followed a first pregnancy and many patients were premature (many weighed only 40 oz. at birth). He noticed the frequency of low intelligence, fits, and uncontrollable behaviour, and the value of massage, baths, gymnastics, and manipulations. He describes a case of marked improvement in an athetoid.

In 1862 Little wrote in an obstetric publication on the influence of abnormal parturition, difficult labour, premature birth, and asphyxia neonatorum on the mental and physical condition of the child, especially in relation to deformities. His description was in many ways in agreement with modern findings, and he mentions for instance that laryngismus stridulus may be present in infancy in these cases, a finding which has only recently been reaffirmed (Apley, 1953). Little states : " Treatment based upon physiology and rational therapeutics effects an amelioration surprising to those who have not watched these cases ". A drawing from this book is shown in the frontispiece.

One or two earlier writers had described cases of cerebral palsy—Collier (1924) quotes Andey (1741), Delpech (1828), and Heine (1860). Little quotes Joerg (1828) as saying that

" too early and unripe born fœtuses may present a state of weakness and stiffness in the muscles persisting until puberty and later ".

Since Little's day there have been numerous articles dealing with specific sides of the subject. As cerebral palsy is the name given to a wide variety of clinical conditions, all the articles are of importance in understanding the complete nature of the condition and not all can be mentioned in any survey.

In 1895 Brissaud thought that prematurity at birth was the causal factor and considered that the essential pathology in symmetrical spastic cases was a lack of complete development of the pyramidal tract—an interesting theory which may contain some truth.

In 1885 Sarah McNutt wrote a paper on cerebral palsy giving clinical details and post-mortem findings in one case which showed meningeal hæmorrhage from pial vessels and venous sinuses, and suggested that this was the essential pathology.

In 1888 Gowers, in an article in *The Lancet*, was strongly of the opinion that most cases were due to cerebral damage at birth, and headed his article " Birth Palsies ". He states that " mental deficiency is not necessarily allied to the muscular disorder ; nor when it exists is there any necessary proportion between the two ". He says that the condition of birth palsy is not uncommon.

In 1889 Osler wrote on *The Cerebral Palsies of Children* from cases he had observed in hospital and in institutions for the feeble-minded. His group of 151 cases included 120 hemiplegics, and he considered a further 20 to be bilateral hemiplegics. Some of his cases were undoubtedly acquired cerebral palsies and he found a high incidence of feeble-mindedness.

Freud (1897) in a monograph discusses 53 cases of bilateral affection. He considered the aetiology of generalized spasticity to be one-third difficult birth and one-sixth premature birth.

Following these early papers, Collier, at the beginning of the century, had an immense influence on the thought given to problems of cerebral palsy and wrote papers in 1899 and 1924. His cases tended to be severe, and over a period of years he came to the conclusion that " the essential anatomical cause of diplegia is a primary degeneration of cerebral neurons from causes which are at present elusive ". The cases he describes and the histories of post-mortem cases give the impression of having been of the type we might now consider rigidities.

Following this early period when various writers came to widely differing conclusions about the aetiology of cerebral palsy, specialists in various branches have investigated the problem as it appeared in their own speciality.

Pathologists examined the brains of cases that died after a history of neurological abnormality dating from birth. Unfortunately most of these cases have been from mental deficiency institutions. There is little evidence that intelligent symmetrical spastic cases have come to post-mortem.

The various pathological surveys have included work by Schwartz (1924, 1927), who showed the frequency of multiple intracerebral hæmorrhages and softenings which occurred especially in the periventricular drainage area of the tributaries of the vein of Galen and considered that these earlier birth lesions led to later porencephaly or sclerosis. Stewart (1942), after examining 50 brains of spastic aments, found diverse lesions, and thought that primary demyelinization explained some lesions, but accepted the possibility that others might be due to anoxia or nutritional deficiencies. As the result of his studies, Courville (1950) considers that many central nervous system degenerative diseases of early and adult life are late results of ante- or intra- or neonatal asphyxia (in addition to cases of infantile cerebral palsy). Throughout this survey we have had the invaluable help of Dr. R. S. Norman (Bristol), who has carried out many post-mortem studies in cases of cerebral palsy and contributed many well-known articles.

Malamud (1950) confirmed the findings of other workers that a condition of *état marbré* in the corpus striatum was found post mortem in cases of athetosis, and suggested that with an intact pyramidal tract cases of *état marbré* with additional damage to the thalamus could give athetosis and idiocy.

These findings of abnormal cerebral pathology in aments who frequently give a history of birth abnormality has led to several investigations of stillbirths and neonatal deaths to see if there is any evidence of brain injury which might have accounted for the early deaths. One of the earliest surveys was by Holland (1922), who examined 300 infants. He found tentorial tears in 75 per cent of dead fœtuses, with damage or kinking of the vein of Galen, and he describes in detail the mechanism of delivery which may cause this.

Various types of intracranial hæmorrhage were noted in these early deaths by Capon (1922). Greenwood (1924), Cruikshank (1930), and the Report No. 94 of the Ministry of Health on Neonatal Mortality and Morbidity (1949) gave figures of various investigations varying from 17 per cent to 55 per cent of the incidence of intracranial hæmorrhage in stillbirths.

Grontoft (1953) found intracranial hæmorrhage in 53 per cent of premature infant deaths and 45 per cent of full-time neonatal deaths, and considered the hæmorrhage was due to asphyxia giving venous congestion in vessels whose walls had been already damaged by hypoxia. He explained the frequency of intraventricular hæmorrhage in prematures, a finding noted by Craig in 1938.

These two findings of cerebral pathology in aments and cerebral damage in neonates have stimulated longitudinal studies into the progress of children who survive various birth abnormalities. There have been follow-ups of prematurity. Ylppö (1922) reported that 7·4 per cent of immature children were idiots or imbeciles and 3·1 per cent had Little's disease. Drillien (1948), who carried out a follow-up in Edinburgh, makes no reference to a spastic case. There appear to be no figures at present to show the proportion of cases of cerebral palsy in each birth-weight group of premature cases—a very necessary investigation in view of the incidence of symmetrical spastic paralysis in low-weight premature babies, as shown later.

Longitudinal studies on neonatal asphyxia have led to varying reports. A résumé of all the surveys was given in a leading article in the *British Medical Journal* (1951), quoting the work of Faber (1947); Belnap, McKhann, and Beck (1950); Rosenfield and Bradley (1948), who also took an interest in the asphyxia of pertussis ; Preston (1945), who took an interest in behaviour disorders ; Keith and Norval (1950) ; and Campbell, Cheeseman, and Kilpatrick (1950). *The overall evidence shows that after neonatal asphyxia cases of cerebral palsy, mental deficiency, fits, behaviour disorders, and learning difficulties do occur, but* THE MAJORITY GROW UP TO BE NORMAL HEALTHY CHILDREN.

Follow-ups of known cases of neonatal cerebral irritation have been carried out by Munro (1928), Capon (1922), and a full survey of 593 cases by Craig (1950), who found later evidence of cerebral palsy in 41 cases, of which 17 were hemiplegics.

In conjunction with the longitudinal studies in birth trauma, many workers have carefully analysed all the cases that they have seen, including antenatal history, birth history, age of mother, parity, etc. These findings tend to vary according to the source of the material. There has been a tendency for the cases to be the severe ones as they were seen in hospital practice, institutions, or at interviews for special school placement. E. S. Evans (1946) saw the cases for admission to Queen Mary's Hospital, Carshalton, and found 10 per cent of the athetoids and more than 60 per cent of the spastics ineducable.

P. R. Evans (1948) gave an account of 114 cases seen in private practice and for admission to a special school. He found a higher incidence of athetoids than usually reported, possibly because this type of case needs special educational placement. McGovern and Yannet (1947) in America felt after a careful examination of 86 cases that the genetic factor was of importance. Dunsdon (1951) carried out a survey in this country for the Ministry of Education and formed a low opinion of the general educability of the cerebral palsied child and discouraged the widespread formation of special educational units.

Of special interest are the surveys carried out in particular districts, which are a serious attempt to examine and analyse all the cases in an area. Asher and Schonell (1950, Birmingham), Holoran (1952, Leeds), Gordon and Scott-Pearson (1949, Belfast), Smallwood (1953, Bristol), and Ingram (1955 a, Edinburgh) have now produced their findings. They tend to use different terminology, but the overall findings are very similar and the total incidence in each area is found to be either just below or just above 2 per 1000.

No account of the literature on cerebral palsy would be representative without mentioning the great masters in America who have made cerebral palsy their particular interest for periods of up to 25 years. Phelps, who has seen about 60,000 cases, has written numerous articles, and many of his original findings, such as sensory loss in spastics and deafness in athetoids (1941), have been confirmed later by other writers. He is primarily an orthopædic surgeon and has taken particular notice of the local bone and muscle defects which may develop in cerebral palsy. Another pædiatrician, Perlstein, has taken an interest in athetosis and speech disorders, whilst Temple Fay has introduced the idea that the movement pattern in cerebral palsy, as for instance the persistent tonic neck reflexes, are a return to an embryological pattern, reptilian and amphibian, and from these observations he has developed some fresh ideas on physiotherapy. Bronson Crothers has written specifically about the total adaptation and psychological needs of the child. He has stressed the value of the environment and of sense training and makes little use of special apparatus, physiotherapy, or surgery. Byers, working in Boston with Bronson Crothers, has taken a particular interest in hemiplegias and in the primitive reflexes of these children. All these five masters have recently visited England. Ford is frequently referred to in the present book, as his large text-book on *Diseases of the Nervous System in Infancy and Childhood* (1944) gives an overall picture of all neurological conditions in childhood and reference to it has revealed the possible conditions we have not yet seen. Lastly, Carlson has stimulated an interest in the subject by his own personality, as he is himself cerebral palsied.

For the full understanding of the neurological abnormalities in these children, contribution by the great English neurologists must form part of the literature. Sherrington's masterpiece, *The Integrative Action of the Nervous System* (1906), is a foundation for all knowledge of reflexes. Kinnier Wilson (1925), Riddoch and Buzzard (1921), and Walshe (1923) in the early 1920s described the primitive reflex patterns in adult cerebral palsies such as hemiplegia and paraplegia. Although these articles are on adult medicine, many of their observations are of direct application to congenital cases. Recently Wyllie has written at length on cerebral palsies, and in particular on acute infantile hemiplegia (1948). During this survey the work of Macdonald Critchley (1953) on parietal lobes has been found particularly interesting, as the symptoms of parietal lobe involvement which he has studied in adults fit very closely the learning difficulties and ' body-image ' upsets of our children in the Bristol Spastic School, and this work has thrown light on many of the educational difficulties that are being encountered.

There have also been several articles on special methods of diagnosis. Electro-encephalographic findings in infantile cerebral palsy have been discussed by Perlstein, Gibbs, and Gibbs (1946) ; air-encephalographic findings by Crothers and Wyatt (1941) ; the radiological diagnosis of subdural hæmatoma by Bull (1949) and Childe (1953). Other articles on special clinical entities such as hereditary spastic palsies, absent corpus callosum, post-measles encephalitis, and sequelæ of prophylactic inoculation are mentioned elsewhere in the text.

Compared with the wide and interesting literature on various aspects of cerebral palsy the literature on treatment, apart from brain surgery, has tended to be slight. Much of it has been written by therapists. The American workers have tended to make use of callipers, walking aids, and other accessory aids. In England there is a growing tendency to dispense with these and treat the child by teaching him the normal movements of an ordinary child in the correct order and pattern, e.g., rolling over, crawling, and walking. To Mrs. Collis, physiotherapist at Queen Mary's Hospital, Carshalton, must be given the credit of introducing the method, although it may have been followed unofficially by parents and children for years. She uses ordinary chairs, spoons, tricycles, etc. Bobath and Bobath have carried this idea of developing normal movement patterns still further by trying to correct the abnormal reflex patterns. If the child has a tonic neck reflex at an age when it should not be there, they try to prevent it. If the child has no *Sprungbereitschaft* or readiness to jump at an age when he should have it, they try to teach it to the child, at the same time trying to overcome abnormal spasm.

Other writers have written excellent monographs on simple treatment which can be carried out at home—Girard (1937), Egel (1948), Pohl (1950). Several writers have taken a particular interest in the teaching of speech to cerebral palsied children (Cass, 1951 ; Palmer, 1952). Others have discussed the treatment of the eyes (Guibor, 1950), or the hand movements and 'methods of grasping' (Hadra, 1950), and recently methods to help learning difficulties (Albitreccia and Tournay, 1954).

Lastly, to understand the defective movement patterns of cerebral palsied children, a study is necessary of normal movement in healthy children. McGraw (1943) has written a simple illustrated book on the baby's normal progress to walking. Byers (1948) has noted the normal reflex patterns of babies, and Weisz (1938) has written on the balance reactions. Steindler (1935) has studied normal and pathological loco-motion with electrical reactions.

Gesell and Amatruda (1949) and Griffiths (1954) have shown the normal skills of babyhood. With the picture of a normal child in mind, a therapist can form a sound basis for work on a cerebral palsied child.

CHAPTER III

THE CLINICAL EXAMINATION

EACH child was seen by a team of workers which consisted of a psychologist, who was the chief educational psychologist of the Bristol Child Guidance Clinic, and thus had immediate contact with the children in school and an easy contact with the educational psychologists in the country areas around ; a school medical officer, who acted as psychiatric social and educational adviser ; and a health visitor, who acted as clinic sister and also contacted the health visitor or school nurse interested in a particular child ; and finally myself, who carried out the full medical examination.

In the medical interview a full family and birth history with details of the antenatal and neonatal period and the birth process was taken. The birth histories were checked wherever possible, although early notes were not always available and sometimes little mention was made of the baby's condition. The age of passing all the milestones, sitting up, crawling, talking, toilet training, were noted and the age at which the mother first suspected that something was wrong. A record was made of illnesses, particularly fits, and of the incidence and dates of immunizations and vaccinations, and whether they had caused any clinical disturbance.

Before the full examination, with the child undressed, the extent of the movement defect was noted—the ability to sit up, roll over, and crawl, and the way in which these actions were done. The importance of noticing upsets in the normal appearance and disappearance of normal infantile reflexes was gradually learned. No attempt was made to analyse the condition of tone in individual muscles as it was early realized that the condition of hypertonicity, spasticity, and even flaccidity was not constant in one group of muscles and certainly not in one muscle, but varied from one muscle group to the other according to the position of the child. Any fixed abnormality such as a contracture or dislocation or subluxation was noted.

A full neurological examination is very difficult in children, particularly babies, and the normal examination of tendon reflexes, etc., is not very helpful. Usually the reflexes were exaggerated in spasticity owing to the stretch reflex, but not in cases of severe spasm amounting to contracture. The abdominal reflexes were usually present, although absent in some hereditary and spinal cases. The plantar reflex was of doubtful value. In cases of severe spasm in the calf muscles, dorsiflexion may be so poor that the reflex is negative. Also if the movement pattern has been altered by operation on the tendo achillis, or on the foot, the reflex may be upset. On the whole, it was found to be extensor in spastics and flexor in athetoids and rigidities.

An attempt was made to analyse the varying defects of vision, hearing, speech, and sensation.

Each child was also seen by the psychologist, who tested the children on whatever scale appeared appropriate. One of the prior duties of the Assessment Team was to make a decision for the Bristol Education Authorities as to the most suitable school for the child. This was a happy arrangement as it meant that a definite numerical I.Q. need not necessarily be obtained. The division was, therefore, made into the groups ineducable, educationally subnormal, normal, superior intelligence. With the additional knowledge of the child's physical handicap, after conference by the team, the school placement was decided. Numerical I.Q.s were only given where definite. With babies arrangements were made for them to be seen every six to nine months by the psychologist, and their intelligence was judged by the progress they were making in social adjustment and response to their environment. Recently the Griffiths scale has been used.

After examination arrangements were made for further investigations—ophthalmological opinion, otological opinion, audiogram, X-ray examination, skull and whole spine, and the urine test for phenylpyruvic acid. E.E.G. records were obtained where possible.

Arrangements were then made, if necessary, for physio-therapy, speech therapy, and occupational therapy, and sometimes remedial coaching.

In some cases, where the diagnosis was in doubt or when fuller investigation was desirable, particularly in the presence of fits, the child was admitted to hospital under a consultant. Air-encephalographic studies were made in 47 cases.

Following these investigations, the children have been seen frequently at a follow-up clinic and any examinations not possible the first time were made at the next or subsequent visits. Records of progress could be made as quite a number of these children have been known to me over many years—some as long as 14 years—and records of their improvement are very interesting.

Finally, special attention was paid to the children at the Bristol School for Spastics. They were the subject of more detailed observations on movement, visual, and hearing defects. These children were particularly studied for evidence of learning or perceptual difficulties.

CHAPTER IV

INCIDENCE OF CEREBRAL PALSY

As the figures of incidence of cerebral palsy from various areas vary fairly considerably, it is possible that different workers are using different assessments of cerebral palsy. Pure cases of spasticity and athetosis are easily noticed, but on the other hand there are many cases of mild cerebral palsy in children attending normal school. Some cases of hemiplegia, particularly on the left side, may be so slight that even the teacher in charge of the child's class may not have noted it. Some cases of athetosis may be considered only fidgety and some ataxic cases may appear to be clumsy. It is often only when an additional symptom, such as a fit or mental backwardness, occurs, that the possibility of cerebral palsy is raised, and then often a history of a premature or difficult birth with neonatal symptoms is obtained and suggests the diagnosis. Because of the interest in Bristol in cerebral palsy, many of these mild cases have been referred to the Cerebral Palsy Assessment Clinic through the Child Guidance Clinic or the School Health Department. The finding of quite a number of these mild cases has undoubtedly weighted the Bristol figures as regards total numbers and has also possibly raised the average intelligence quotient of cerebral palsied cases to a higher figure than is usually given. In quite a number of cases referred to the clinic, however, there has been no neurological evidence of cerebral palsy, and the condition has been thought to be either constitutional or emotional and the cases have not been included. There is sometimes, though, a history of difficult birth and mental backwardness and the possible significance of the combination requires further elucidation.

In *Table I* the occurrence of the Bristol cases in each year of birth is noted. A case has been taken to be a Bristol case if the child was resident in Bristol at the time of the examination.

There is, of course, some coming and going between Bristol and outside areas, but it is taken for granted that as many move in as move out. This may be a slight fallacy, as a few parents have purposely moved into Bristol to obtain more adequate education for their handicapped child. On the whole it seems fair to compare the total number of cases in the years 1938–50 with the total live births in those years.

Table I.—INCIDENCE IN BRISTOL

Year	Paraplegia	Monoplegia	Hemiplegia	Quadriplegia	Athetosis	Ataxia	Rigidity	Total	Premature	Live Births
1936 and earlier	1	—	6	4	—	—	—	11	7	
1937	—	1	—	2	—	—	—	3	1	
1938	2	2	3	3	2	1	—	13	3	6058
1939	1	2	4	2	—	1	—	10	2	6219
1940	—	—	2	—	—	1	—	3	1	6363
1941	1	1	2	1	—	2	—	7	1	5379
1942	—	—	7	2*	1	—	2	12	—	6422
1943	2	—	1	2	—	—	—	5	2	6885
1944	2	—	6	3	—	2	3	16	6	7767
1945	—	—	7	4	2	2	1	16	4	7027
1946	2	—	5	3*	4	—	1	15	4	8041
1947	—	2	5	5	2	5	3	22	7	9142
1948	2	1	13	3	2	—	1	25	5	7831
1949	1	1	6	3	3	3	4	21	7	7506
1950	1	1	3	1	2	2	1	11	2	7096
1951	—	1	4	1	2	1	2	11	4	6872
1952	2	—	5	2	1	—	2	12	4	6760
1953	—	—	—	1	1	—	—	2	—	6945
1954	—	—	—	3 (seen later)	1	—	—	1	1	6691
								216		

* 1 died.

After 1950 the figures are not yet likely to be complete. Included in the list are cases of cerebral palsy deaths, so that from this table we can obtain the figures of the average number of cerebral palsy children who reached 5 years of age per 1000 live births in the years 1938–51. The figure is 1·90.

As will be seen from *Table I*, there is an apparent increase in cases in all groups in the years 1947, 1948, 1949. Some of this increase is due to a bulge in the birth-rate in those years ;

it is reflected in the larger number of live births in the years shown. From the year 1947 onwards the premature baby service has been active in saving the lives of tiny premature babies, but from the figures premature births account for only a fraction of the total increase in cerebral palsy cases. The possible reason may be that in many families the mother was having her first baby after the war years and there tended to be a larger number of older mothers and a larger number of them having their first baby.

In *Table II* the percentage incidence of the various types of movement upset is given both for the Bristol cases and for the whole survey. As will be seen, there is a higher incidence of hemiplegias and monoplegias in the Bristol cases.

Table II.—PERCENTAGE INCIDENCE OF DIFFERENT TYPES

Movement Defect	Bristol Cases		Outside Cases		Whole Survey	
	No.	Per cent	No.	Per cent	No.	Per cent
Paraplegia ..	17	7·9	9	10·5	26	8·2
Monoplegia ..	12	5·6	1	1·2	13	4·1
Hemiplegia ..	79	36·6	18	21·2	97	32·7
Quadriplegia ..	42	19·4	33	38·8	75	24·9
Athetosis ..	24	11·1	9	10·5	33	10·9
Ataxia ..	23	10·6	6	7·1	29	9·6
Rigidity ..	19	8·8	9	10·5	28	9·3
	216		85		301	

Almost certainly the reason for this is that hemiplegias and monoplegias fit into normal schools and therefore have not so readily been referred to the Assessment Team from the areas around.

The Bristol figures can thus be considered a fairly accurate enumeration of the various types of cerebral palsy in the total population. As already stated, in this investigation into aetiological and clinical signs of cerebral palsy the total number of cases in each category is considered as a whole. It was felt that no useful purpose would be served by separating the Bristol and outside-Bristol cases when discussing clinical signs.

Summary.—From the Bristol figures the number of cerebral palsied children who reach the age of 5 years is 1·90 per 1000 live births.

CHAPTER V

PARAPLEGIA

IN subdividing the cases of cerebral palsy under headings which describe only the upset of movement pattern, the first group for discussion is the spastic paraplegias. Twenty-six cases have been seen and the degree of spasticity and movement upset varies from case to case, but tends to follow the pattern originally described by Little.

The movement defect varies according to whether the child is in extension, lying supine, or attempting to stand, or whether the child is in flexion, sitting, or crawling. In extension there is extension, adduction, and internal rotation of the hips, with partial extension of the knees and plantar flexion of the feet, giving the scissors appearance. This is the typical appearance that is produced by holding the child up by support under the arms. In flexion there is flexion and abduction of the hips with flexion of the knees and dorsiflexion of the ankles.

All these positions of the joints are caused by spasticity in the muscle group concerned. The abnormality of tone in the muscles can be revealed, for example, by attempting to flex the hip or knee when the child is trying to stand, or to extend the knee when the child is sitting.

Thus, a paraplegic child who attempts to walk before the abnormal tone in the muscles has been corrected by treatment will develop the typical scissors gait. Contrarily, the paraplegic child who spends long periods sitting in a chair will develop severe flexor deformities of the hips and knees.

Again, the paraplegic child who attempts to walk too early will walk with severe extension of the hips and spine. In order that the child can look forward, he will learn to flex his head at the atlanto-occipital joint and walk with an odd ' poked forward ' appearance. This abnormality is shown in *Fig.* 1. It is suggested that this abnormal posture may account for the cases of apparent dislocation of the atlanto-occipital joint that have been noted in adult cases by Temple Fay (unpublished lecture at Bristol School for Spastics, 1954).

All these 26 cases have been placed under the separate heading of spastic paraplegia because there was no typical spasticity in the hands and upper limbs. However, more severe cases of paraplegia, with a certain amount of spine and shoulder involvement, appear to blend into cases of spastic quadriplegia with arm involvement, and as will be shown later, the aetiology of these two types of spastic motor upset may be similar. In fact, in some of the severe cases of spastic paraplegia there is an unusual clumsiness of the hand movements which might be due to minimal spasticity.

Again, at the other end of the scale, very mild cases of spastic paraplegia may involve only the legs or feet.

NUMERICAL FINDINGS

Family History.—
　　7 (2 talipes in mother ; 1 abnormal sibling ; 1 cousin ' crippled ' ; 3 similar condition in family).
Mother's Age at Birth.—
　　Under 20, 0 ; 20–30 years, 10 ; 30–40 years, 15 ; over 40 years, 1.
Order of Pregnancy.—
　　First, 11 ; second, 7 ; third, 3 ; fourth, 5.
Gestation Period.—
　　Under 33 weeks, 12 ; 33–38 weeks, 4 ; 39–42 weeks, 10.
Birth Process.—
　　Pre-eclampsia, 4.
　　Other antenatal illness, 15 (including 8 cases of uterine hæmorrhage in pregnancy).
　　Breech, 3 ; Forceps, 1 ; Cæsarean (for pre-eclampsia), 2.
　　Multiple birth, 3.
　　Precipitate birth, 4.
　　Long labour (over 24 hours), 2.
　　Normal full-time birth, 6.
Male : Female : 14 : 12.
Birth Weights.—
　　Under 4 lb., 12 ; 4 lb.+, 2 ; 5 lb.+, 3 ; 6 lb.+, 1 ; 7 lb.+, 4 ; 8 lb.+, 3 ; uncertain, 1. Premature—i.e., 5½ lb. and under, 15.
Neonatal Abnormalities.—
　　Asphyxia, 8 ; Jaundice, 4 ; Cerebral irritation, 3.
*Convulsion after 4 weeks of age.—*5.
*Cerebral Infection in Infancy.—*2.

Vision.—
  Impaired sight, 1.
  Muscular imbalance of eyes, 9.
Hearing Defect.—1.
Speech Defect.—3.
Hand Dominance.—Only 1 definitely left-handed.
Hydrocephalus (i.e., 1 in. above normal for age).—3.
Microcephalus (i.e., 1 in. below normal for age).—2.
I.Q.—Under 50, 5 ; 50–69, 1 ; 70–89, 5 ; 90–109, 9 ; 110–129, 4 ;
    130+, 1 ; Uncertain, 1.
School Placement.—O.S., 10 ; Spastic School, 2 ; P.H.S., 6 ;
    E.S.N., 0 ; Oc.C., 5 ; None at present, 3.

The above figures are only a crude statement of the clinical findings in the cases of paraplegia, and point to the fact that we are not dealing with a single clinical entity, and that the movement pattern defect is only one symptom of the condition. Our findings suggest that these cases can be divided into distinct clinical syndromes of which spastic paraplegia is only one sign.

GROUP 1. HEREDITARY GROUP

The strong family history covers a group of 3 cases in which the condition was undoubtedly genetically determined. There were two sisters with a similar condition, and a boy whose mother was also affected.

The two sisters shown in *Fig.* 2 had a typical spastic paraplegia present from birth, with no history of birth abnormality or evidence of sensory loss, intellectual impairment, or other neurological signs. Their father had a similar condition which had first manifested itself whilst serving during the war. Two paternal aunts were stated to have been affected since birth, and were showing deterioration in adult life. One had given birth to a hydrocephalic infant. Other members of the family were said to be " hen-toed ".

The boy had a less severe affection. His mother, grandfather, great uncle, and two uncles had a similar condition. This boy had been born prematurely, and the cause of his condition had been considered as due to a birth injury until the family history was obtained.

Hereditary cases of spastic paraplegia have been reported by many observers. Dick and Stevenson (1953) describes a family with spastic paraplegia and associated pyramidal symptoms. Schwartz (1952) describes three families with a pure form of hereditary spastic paraplegia, all starting in middle life. Crowe (1944) describes a family with 5 children, all typical paraplegias, with the additional symptom of strabismus. Bickerstaff (1950) gives an account of a family with spastic paraplegia and other signs of neurological abnormality, in which the symptoms appeared earlier in each generation. He says that the various " hereditary familial disorders of the nervous system are inter-related ". In this connexion the occurrence of a case of hydrocephalus in the first family described might be of interest.

These cases raise the possibility that other cases of paraplegia or also of cerebral palsy may be hereditary. At least two other cases of paraplegia in this series are ' under suspicion '. Two other mothers gave a history of talipes as babies and possibly this condition could be related. In Bickerstaff's family one case showed marked pes cavus.

GROUP 2. PARAPLEGIA FOLLOWING PREMATURITY

Prematurity appears to be the most remarkable factor in the second group of cases. No less than 15 of the 26 cases of paraplegia were premature, and of these 11 were under 4 lb. in weight at birth, of which 8 again were 3 lb. or under. As 13 of these cases tended to be similar clinically, the prematurity by itself must be a significant factor, and be a guide to the understanding of the pathology.

These 13 children were born after an unusually short gestation period, and the reason for this appeared to be ante-partum hæmorrhage (including threatened miscarriage) in 6 cases, and in 2 cases a severe pre-eclampsia necessitating early induction of labour.

Following a premature birth, there is usually a fairly difficult neonatal period with signs of shallow respiration, œdema, jaundice, feeding difficulty, and, quite frequently, twitching and other signs of cerebral irritation. These symptoms were reported in quite a number of these tiny premature babies, who later developed spasticity. In view of the fact that these symptoms are shown even to a severe degree in a premature baby who later develops quite normally, the significance of a stormy neonatal period is difficult to assess. In contrast, some of our paraplegic cases showed surprisingly little neonatal disturbance. In 3 cases, however, neonatal jaundice was particularly severe.

From a survey of the cases that follow it would appear that severe prematurity by itself was the overriding factor in the later manifestation of spastic paraplegia, but that in a few cases there had been additional brain damage—a natural hazard of a premature birth.

The movement upset in these 13 children showed all degrees of severity.

In the mildest case—a twin, birth-weight 2 lb.—there was a spastic pes cavus, with very slight spasticity of the calf muscles and a tendency to walk in equinus (*Fig.* 3). It is suggested that the marked pes cavus with plantar extensor responses represents a very mild case of this type.

In the slightly more severe cases, 4 in number, there was spasticity of the calf muscles, with a marked tendency to walk in equinus with flexion at the knee (*Figs.* 4, 5).

Five more severe cases showed, in addition, internal rotation of the hips with knocking of the knees—a mild scissors gait.

In the 3 most severe cases there was also flexion of the hip and compensatory extension of the spine with marked lordosis. In these last cases, the arms were ' under suspicion ' ; thus it is felt that cases of symmetrical quadriplegia with a history of premature birth may be an extension of this group (*Fig.* 6).

No sensory defects were noted. The abdominal reflexes were always present, and the plantar reflexes extensor, except in the presence of contractures of the calf muscles, with corresponding flaccidity of the dorsiflexors. The X-ray examination of the spine has been normal in the 10 cases taken.

The E.E.G. has been normal in 10 cases, of a ' quiet ' type in 1, and suggestive of convulsions in 2. The I.Q.s were within normal limits in 12 cases, but one child was ineducable. This child was the only one having fits, and had impaired vision and an abnormal E.E.G. An air-encephalogram was normal in one case and in another (the other child with an abnormal E.E.G.) showed dilatation of the posterior half of the left lateral ventricle consistent with cerebral atrophy.

An interesting additional sign in this group is a muscular imbalance of the eyes, with a tendency to convergence. This was present from birth in 7 cases. This must be considered an associated movement defect. Dunsdon (1951) noted an incidence of strabismus in 33 per cent of her paraplegic cases— a higher figure of strabismus than in her other groups and a finding she could not explain.

Thus in this group there were 11 children with normal intelligence whose only handicap was a spastic paraplegia, and in some cases an eye movement defect ; and 2 similar children who showed evidence of additional brain damage, 1 ineducable microcephalic epileptic, and 1 with an abnormal air-encephalogram and electro-encephalogram.

The outstanding feature is the symmetrical nature of the lesion, which makes it difficult to guess at the pathology. There is no clear evidence that a case of this type has come to post-mortem. It has been suggested that a symmetrical venous damage, either hæmorrhagic or thrombotic, may have occurred in veins draining into the longitudinal sinus, which would cause damage to the leg areas. This might not account for the high incidence of eye defects. It has been shown by Craig (1938) that a typical lesion in stillborn premature babies is an intraventricular hæmorrhage. In a survivor this might cause cerebral atrophy and associated enlargement of the lateral ventricles. If the cerebral damage was anteriorly, this could affect the leg and eye muscle areas. On the other hand, the original suggestion by Brissaud (1895) that the pyramidal tracts in the premature baby have not fully matured may be correct. At the age of 6 months of intra-uterine life they have only reached the cervical areas, and the lumbar region by the 7th–8th months. The extranatal growth of these fibres may be slower or cease altogether, and may give rise to a paraplegia. A possible connexion between these cases and retrolental fibroplasia has been suggested and has been seen in 2 later cases. Obviously until a case of this type comes to pathological investigation, the true cerebral abnormality will not be known.

Thus, in this series of 26 cases of spastic paraplegia, 12 appear to group themselves into a loosely defined group of severe prematurity with normal intelligence. There was evidence of further brain damage in 1 case.

GROUP 3. PARAPLEGIA FOLLOWING BIRTH TRAUMA

The aetiology of 4 cases of spastic paraplegia appeared to be some cerebral catastrophe during the birth process ; and an additional sign which links these 4 cases is hydrocephalus.

One hyperexcitable mentally defective child was born after a long labour and forceps delivery. He showed a mild spastic paraplegia, with a tendency to walk on tip-toe, and a moderate degree of hydrocephalus.

A further child had white asphyxia following a forceps delivery and was similar to the child above except that he showed a higher intelligence.

Another child was born after a pregnancy complicated by pre-eclampsia and an A.P.H. There were severe neonatal difficulties. His head was observed to enlarge slowly from infancy and he suffered from fits. He had a spastic paraplegia, and some involvement of the trunk muscles, with a muscular imbalance of the eyes (*Fig.* 7). He was ineducable.

Lastly, a fourth child was born prematurely weighing 3 lb. 3 oz. The hydrocephalus gradually developed from 12 months of age and showed a circumference of 25 in. at 8 years. She had a mild spastic paraplegia and an I.Q. of 89.

The pathology in these cases has been investigated by Yakovlev (1947). He shows that in hydrocephalus a dilatation of the lateral ventricles will stretch the long motor-fibres coming from the upper third of the precentral gyrus, the paracentral lobules, and the posterior third of the superior frontal gyrus, more than the shorter motor-fibres which originate lower down in the lateral wall of the cerebral hemisphere. The former fibres are the pyramidal tract fibres for the lower extremities, and the latter the fibres for the face and upper extremities. Thus, dilatation of the lateral ventricles in hydrocephalus can cause a spasticity of the lower extremities. This pathology may explain these 4 cases of paraplegia coupled with hydrocephalus following a history of birth trauma.

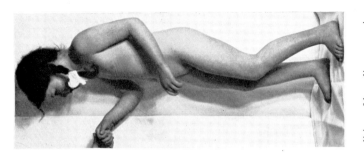

Fig. 1.—A case of severe paraplegia showing the 'poked forward'
appearance of the head.

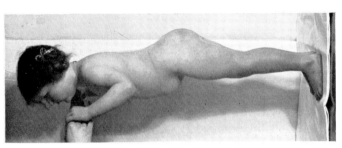

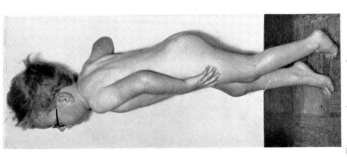

Fig. 2.—Two sisters with the condition of hereditary spastic
paraplegia.

PLATE II

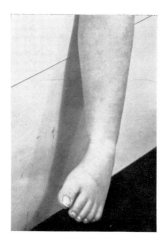

Fig. 3.—Mild pes cavus and spasticity of the calf muscles in a child of 5 years (birth weight 2 lb.).

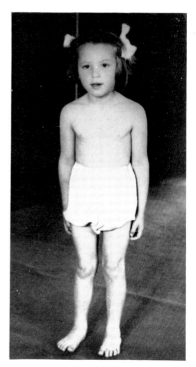

Fig. 4.—A mild case of spastic paraplegia (birth weight 3 lb.). She learnt to walk at 3½ years of age.

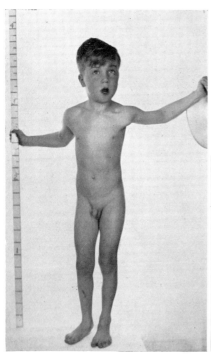

A

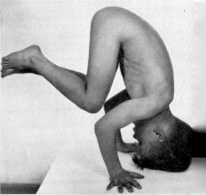

B

Fig. 5.—A, A case of spastic paraplegia (birth weight 3 lb.). B, His ability to s on his hands demonstrates the fact that his arms are not affected.

PLATE III

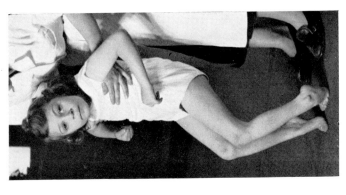

Fig. 8.—A case of spastic paraplegia with sensory loss in the hands.

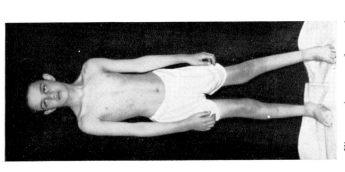

Fig. 7.—A case of spastic paraplegia with hydrocephalus, mental deficiency, and epilepsy.

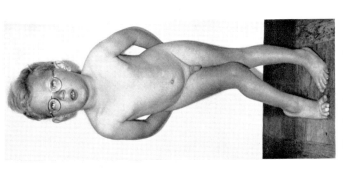

Fig. 6.—A case of severe spastic paraplegia (birth weight 2 lb.). There is some spinal involvement.

PLATE IV

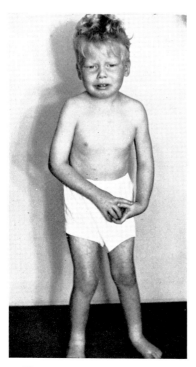

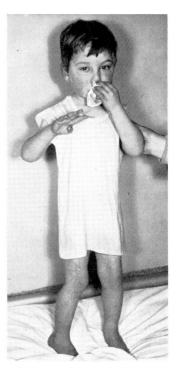

Fig. 9.—A case of left monoplegia with motor aphasia following pertussis at 8 months.

Fig. 10.—A case of right-sided congenital hemiplegia with epilepsy and normal intelligence.

GROUP 4. SPINAL DEFECTS

Possibly the following 2 cases should not be included in a survey on cerebral palsy as they are correctly cases of spinal palsy. However, both presented as cases of cerebral palsy and had for many years been treated and considered as such.

Case 1.—An only child born after a normal birth, weighing 7 lb. 2 oz. The abnormality in his legs was noted from birth. When he was first seen his movement pattern had been altered by a bilateral E.T.A. operation, but he then walked with flexed hips and knees and flat feet. There was evidence of spasticity in the hamstring and hip flexors. His abdominal reflexes were absent. He suffered from urinary incontinence. A spinal radiograph showed a defect between T.4 and T.10, and a myelogram gave some evidence of a bifid cord. He was then considered to be a case of diastomatomyelia.

Case 2.—An only child weighing 9 lb. at birth, born after a normal delivery. He walked at 2 years, and had a gait rather similar to that of the two little girls in the hereditary group. On examination, he had slight general spasticity with patellar and ankle clonus, but his gait appeared slightly ataxic, with flexed hips and knees. There was slight loss of vibration sense and sense of position in the lower limbs. He suffered from diurnal and nocturnal urinary incontinence. The plantar responses were extensor. He could move his eyes up and down, but not inwards and outwards. He had right ear deafness, and there was evidence of spinal defect in his cervical spine. His intelligence was above normal. He was considered to be a case of multiple congenital defects, and it is suggested later that one or two other cases of cerebral palsy may be of this type.

GROUP 5. POST-INFECTIVE PARAPLEGIA

In this group were 2 cases considered by the parents to have followed an attack of meningitis in childhood. In both cases there had been a history of birth difficulty, and it appears doubtful whether they were normal children before the attacks of meningitis. This last finding may be interesting, as in several of the cases of cerebral palsy of all movement upset types, which appeared to be due to a postnatal cause, the evidence was suggestive of developmental abnormality before the causal illness.

Case 3.—Born as the second twin after a gestation period of 37 weeks, weighing 7 lb. at birth. There was slight feeding difficulty only. The school record shows that she was not as ' forward ' as her other twin. There was an attack of meningitis (? type) at 5 years of age. On examination, she was found to have a mild spastic para-plegia with pes cavus. She was microcephalic and ineducable and had an E.E.G. suggestive of petit mal. The paraplegia in this case was minimal ; but the total cerebral damage must have been out of proportion to the movement upset.

Case 4.—Born prematurely after a 30-week gestation period, weighing 5 lb. 4 oz. There were severe neonatal difficulties. She had cerebrospinal meningitis at 4 months of age. On examination at 13½ years, she was found to have severe spastic paraplegia with bilateral upward displacement of the femoral heads, presumably due to the spasticity. She was unable to walk alone. There was a slight tremor in the hands, and hydrocephalus with a circumference of 25 in. was present. She was ineducable and there was gross obesity probably of hypothalamic origin. She had optic atrophy.

GROUP 6. UNKNOWN CAUSES

Finally, there were 2 cases of spastic paraplegia which did not fall clearly into any of the above groups :—

Case 5.—Born precipitately into a bucket, and weighing 6 lb. 2 oz. There were no neonatal symptoms of cerebral damage. He had a severe paraplegia with slight learning difficulties, which will be discussed in a later chapter. His I.Q., E.E.G., A.E.G., and spine radiograph were normal. His general muscle power was poor. There was no significant family history, but his condition strongly suggested a genetic origin.

Case 6.—Born normally, weighing 7 lb. 6 oz., after a pregnancy complicated by a threatened miscarriage. There was a history of an abnormal stillborn sibling. Her spastic condition was particularly severe, and there was some evidence of awkwardness in her hands. On examination, it was interesting to find that she had astereognosis in both hands and showed a Gerstmann's syndrome. She showed interesting learning difficulties. (*Fig.* 8.)

DISCUSSION

In this small series of 26 cases of spastic paraplegia, six distinct clinical types have been noted. From a review of the literature it appears that there are other clinical causes of infantile spastic paraplegia which we have not had the oppor-tunity to see to date.

1. A spastic paraplegia may be due to a spinal birth injury (Ford, 1944). There does not appear to be a case of this type in the Bristol child population ; and it must be a rare happening.

2. Cases may occur as the result of congenital syphilis (Ford). Possibly the thorough antenatal investigation and treatment of all syphilitic mothers has virtually eliminated these cases.

3. Spastic paraplegia may occur after a measles encephalomyelitis (Ford). The 2 cases of cerebral palsy in this survey which appeared to follow measles had involvement of the upper limb in addition to cerebral defects.

SUMMARY

Twenty-six cases of spastic paraplegia are under discussion. The movement defect is described in detail. An attempt has been made to elucidate the aetiology.

The 26 cases appear to fall into six distinct clinical groups.

Three were genetically determined.

In 13 cases the significant feature appeared to be a history of prematurity.

Four cases appeared to follow birth trauma.

Two cases followed postnatal cerebral infection.

Two cases were more correctly cases of spinal palsy and showed congenital spinal defects.

Two cases with unusual sensory defects fell into no particular clinical grouping, and may be genetically determined.

It is suggested that there are other clinical conditions which may lead to infantile spastic paraplegia but which have not been encountered in this survey.

CHAPTER VI

MONOPLEGIA

A FURTHER interesting type of cerebral palsy, comparable in many ways with the paraplegias, was the cases of monoplegia. Thirteen were seen, and again they did not fall into one clinical group. In some cases the nature of the paralysis was spasticity and in other flaccidity, and in all the cases seen one leg only was affected. One or two cerebral palsy cases had originally been considered as examples of spastic monoplegia of an arm only, but on careful examination minimal spasticity in the leg of the same side was noted and the cases were therefore classified as hemiplegia.

The movement upset in all cases seen was slight, and involved the leg and foot, with no evidence of spastic hip flexion, internal rotation, or adduction. In some cases there was extreme spasticity of the calf muscles amounting to contracture, with poor or absent power in the dorsiflexors and marked tendency to walk in equinus. In these cases there was a defect of growth. Owing to the apparently mild nature of the condition in many cases, no demand for treatment had been made and this severe condition had developed. The knee-jerks were obtained in all cases and in most were exaggerated. The plantar response was extensor, except where dorsiflexion was very weak or the architecture of the foot had been altered by operations.

In the 2 flaccid cases, the differential diagnosis was anterior poliomyelitis. There was flaccidity of the leg muscles with slight wasting and pes planus. The jerks, however, were slightly exaggerated. In one case the condition dated from a severe attack of pertussis at 8 months of age and apart from the monoplegia there was a motor aphasia and a suggestion of ataxia (*Fig.* 9). In the other case (*Case* 7) there had been a difficult forceps delivery with neonatal illness.

Case 7.—The child had slight asymmetry of the face, with persistent dribbling and defective speech, an incoordinated gait, and an intelligence below normal.

In both cases the evidence pointed to a cerebral rather than a spinal cause. In no case was there evidence of sensory loss.

The numerical findings, which are too small for statistical analysis, are given below :—

Family History.—
    1 brother spastic died at 7 months ; 1 brother athetoid ; 1 cousin similar condition.

Mother's Age at Birth.—
    20–30 years, 7 ; 30–40 years, 6.

Order of Pregnancy.—
    First, 4 ; second, 5 ; third, 2 ; fourth, 2.

Gestation Period.—
    Under 33 weeks, 4 ; 33–38 weeks, 0 ; 39–42 weeks, 8 ; uncertain, 1.

Birth Process.—
    Pre-eclampsia, slight, 1. Eclampsia, 1.
    Forceps, 1.
    Multiple, 2.
    Precipitate, 1.
    Normal full-time birth, 6.

Male : Female : 6 : 7.

Birth Weights.—
    Under 4 lb., 2 ; 4 lb.+, 1 ; 5 lb.+, 3 ; 6 lb.+, 4 ; 7 lb.+, 3 ;
    Premature, 6.

Neonatal Abnormalities.—
    Asphyxia, 1 ; Jaundice, 1 ; Feeding difficulty, 2.

Associated Congenital Defects.—
    Spina bifida and nystagmus, 1.

*Convulsions.—*2.

*Postnatal Cerebral Infection or Vascular Catastrophe.—*1.

*Muscular Imbalance of Eyes.—*6.

*Hearing Defect.—*0.

*Speech Defect.—*4.

*Hand Dominance.—*3 left (all mentally backward).

*Hydrocephalus.—*1.

*Microcephalus.—*1.

I.Q.—
    Under 50, 1 ; 50–69, 3 ; 70–89, 2 ; 90–109, 2 ; 110–129, 3 ; 130+, 2.

School Placement.—
    O.S., 9 ; E.S.N., 2 ; Spastic School, 1 ; Oc.C., 1.

On analysis, these cases of monoplegia appear to fall into the clinical groups suggested for paraplegia, and it may be that we are dealing with mild cases of the same pathology. They are thus discussed under the same headings.

1. Hereditary.—In 1 case there was a suggestive family history of a cousin with a similar condition. This was a girl born after a normal delivery with an I.Q. of 145. Unfortunately, an E.E.G. and further investigation were refused. The spine radiograph was normal.

2. Prematurity.—As no fewer than 6 of these 13 cases were premature at birth, it must be a significant factor. Three weighed under 4 lb. at birth. As in the group of paraplegics, there was a high incidence of muscular imbalance of the eyes. Three had an internal strabismus and 1 nystagmus. Five had normal or superior intelligence. On the grounds of prematurity, normal intelligence, and no other neurological sign except muscular imbalance of the eyes, one is tempted to wonder if some of these monoplegia cases do not fit into a group with a similar pathology to the premature paraplegics of the previous chapter, and represent only a milder condition. Again, however, there was evidence of additional brain damage in the following case—a hazard of premature birth.

Case 8.—A twin weighing 3 lb. at birth who suffered from severe jaundice and feeding difficulties in the neonatal period. He had a mild left spastic monoplegia with muscular imbalance of the eyes. He suffered from frequent petit mal attacks, confirmed by an E.E.G., and his I.Q. was 65. He attended a school for educationally subnormal children.

3. Birth Trauma.—Birth trauma appears to have been the cause of flaccid monoplegia in *Case* 7 discussed above. Various theories have been advanced as to the pathology of flaccidity of cerebral origin, and in this survey very few cases have been seen. It was suggested by Phelps (1949) that damage to area 4 of the frontal cortex may account for this type of lesion.

The following case may also be due to birth injury ; she suffers from hydrocephalus, which was a prominent symptom in the corresponding paraplegic group.

Case 9.—Born prematurely, weighing 5 lb. 6 oz. There were no neonatal difficulties. She had mild hydrocephalus, with a skull measurement of $21\frac{1}{2}$ in. at $4\frac{1}{2}$ years. There was a right internal strabismus, with a field of vision defect on that side. There was a right spastic monoplegia with poor dorsiflexion. The E.E.G. revealed focal discharges from the right occipital lobe, with liability to epilepsy. Fits have not occurred. Her I.Q. was 108. She was right-handed. Her brother died of fits at 7 years of age, and was said to have been spastic.

4. Multiple Congenital Defects.—One girl with normal intelligence and a right spastic monoplegia had evidence of multiple congenital defects. There was, in addition, congenital nystagmus, an inability to look upwards, and a lumbar meningocele which had been operated on at birth. This could hardly have accounted for the spastic monoplegia. The rest of the spine was normal radiologically. She may be comparable to *Case* 2 in the paraplegic group.

5. Cerebral Catastrophe in Infancy.—This appeared to be the causal factor in one case.

Case 10.—The second child, born after a normal birth, weighing 8 lb. His mother considered that he was a normal baby until a severe attack of pertussis at 8 months of age. Soon afterwards a flaccid paralysis was noted in the left leg. At 3 years of age he gave the impression of a miserable immature child with no speech and inability to walk. The knee-jerks were present and the plantar reflexes equivocal. There was ½ in. wasting and shortening of the leg. Radiographs of the spine, skull, and pelvis were normal. An air-encephalogram was normal. He was admitted to a Spastic School at 4 years and was then able to walk. His walk was incoordinated and on a wide base. He still had no speech, but he obviously understood all that was said to him and reacted intelligently, even politely, to situations. It was felt that he may be suffering from a motor aphasia, and is now receiving speech therapy. Presumably the original catastrophe was asphyxial or vascular in nature.

6. Unknown Cause.—One feeble-minded boy, seen in this survey, had a right spastic monoplegia, with some evidence of ataxia, internal strabismus, and impaired vision due to optic atrophy. The birth was normal and the cause of the condition was obscure.

A spastic monoplegia was also found in a normal little school-child of average intelligence. No cause for the condition was elucidated.

DISCUSSION

These interesting cases of monoplegia show again a hetero-geneous collection of clinical types, and this attempt to put them under distinct headings must only be hypothetical. In most of the cases the evidence that there was cerebral damage appears to be strong. Ford (1944) states that usually monoplegia is due to birth injury. He also states that if only one limb is affected the cerebral damage or defect must be at a cortical level.

It has also been suggested that monoplegia may be due to syphilis, tuberculoma, or cerebral tumour (Ford). Examples of these types were not met with in this small group.

This series of cases emphasizes the fact that the amount of upset of movement pattern does not correspond with the total cerebral disorientation. In this series one child was mentally defective and two educationally subnormal—one with fits—despite the relative insignificance of the palsy.

SUMMARY

Thirteen cases of spastic monoplegia have been seen, in every case involving one leg.

The aetiology appears to be similar to that of spastic paraplegia.

One case was genetically determined.

Six gave a history of prematurity, with additional evidence of birth trauma in one case.

Two cases followed birth trauma.

One followed a severe pertussis infection at 8 months.

One showed multiple congenital defects.

One mentally defective boy and one normally intelligent child did not fall into any definite aetiological group.

Other clinical conditions which may give rise to spastic monoplegia are mentioned.

CHAPTER VII

HEMIPLEGIA

THIS group of cases is of interest and importance, both because of the large number and also because of the existence of this condition among the normal school population and working adult population. The majority of the children in this group attended normal school and were making a good to fair adjustment (*Fig.* 10). In some cases the disability had not been noted by the class teacher. By close liaison with the Bristol School Health Service, which is responsible for the periodic medical inspection of schoolchildren, possibly all the children with spastic hemiplegia in the school population were seen, and the total survey shows some very interesting findings—in particular the occurrence of a fair number of hemiplegics of above normal, or even superior, intelligence. It has been stated by Stewart (1948) that " mental deficiency in some degree is present in a large proportion of cases " ; by McIntire (1947) that 25 per cent were either idiots or imbeciles ; and by Collis (1954) that in " hemiplegics there were usually signs of mental abnormality and speech retardation ". Only 9 in our series of 95 were considered ineducable, and the comparative intelligence of the right and left hemiplegics given later is particularly interesting.

Spastic hemiplegia is a movement defect affecting one side of the body only. Occasionally a case, previously diagnosed as hemiplegia, was found to have minimal involvement of the other side—a slight spasticity or mild athetoid movement, or a pes cavus or pes planus of neurological origin—and the case was referred to the group of quadriplegics. One case, which showed a severe speech disorder due to bilateral spasticity of the tongue and face muscles, was found on examination to have minimal involvement on the other side, and bilateral cerebral damage was confirmed by air encephalography.

As with all other movement-defect groups, the abnormality was not uniform, and wide variations in the basic handicap were noted. The arm was always more severely affected than the leg. This may be due to the fact that the leg must be used in walking, whereas the child can get on quite well using only one arm.

In the typical case the defect is one of fairly severe spasticity. The upper limb is held with the arm adducted and internally rotated, the forearm flexed and pronated, the wrists flexed, and the fingers flexed with the thumb pressed against the palm. Unless the child is encouraged to use the limb, contractures develop in the elbow and wrist flexors and the forearm pronators, and the limb is fixed permanently in this position. On passive movement the leg shows little abnormality at the hips and adductor spasm is not usually noted. There is severe spasticity of the calf muscles, and the foot is held in plantar flexion. Dorsiflexion of the foot is always weak in hemiplegia, unless practised very adequately and from an early age. The spasm in the calf muscles may lead to permanent contractures.

Because of the poor dorsiflexion the child tends to walk with the heel raised. There is also a spasm in the trunk muscles of the affected side. Both these factors cause the child to abduct the hip and swing the lower limb. Eventually the leg may appear shorter than its fellow and in some cases this apparent defect in growth is caused by spasticity in the trunk muscles of that side, and could be prevented by overcoming the spasm of the trunk muscles and encouraging active dorsiflexion. The spasm in the trunk muscles can produce a scoliosis. The lower part of the face and the tongue may be affected and there may be an internal strabismus on the affected side.

Dorsiflexion of the foot is often easier to perform with the knee flexed. This has been thought to be due to the persistence of the flexor withdrawal reflex. The extreme plantar flexion in the extended or upright position is considered to be a reflex standing posture and, as shown by Walshe (1923), Riddoch and Buzzard (1921), part of the pattern of decerebrate rigidity.

In the majority of cases, so-called associated movements are present. When the child makes a strong muscular movement with his non-affected limb, the affected side partially or completely assumes the typical hemiplegic position. Walshe has shown that these associated movements are primitive reflex movements released because the limb is no longer under cortical control, and are " postural reactions allied to tonic reflexes and decerebrate rigidity ". There is evidence of a symmetrical tonic neck reflex in associated movements.

These associated movements must be a serious handicap to the child. One intelligent adult told me that she could hold a cup and saucer in her affected hand, but if she then stirred her tea with a spoon held in the non-affected hand, her hemiplegic hand went into spasm and she dropped the cup and saucer. One normal boy found that he could not play football by standing on his affected leg and kicking with his normal leg, as the affected leg let him down. He therefore kicked with his affected leg held in a stiff extended position, and gave considerable strain and pain to his abdominal muscles. Work in the gymnasium may be more difficult for these children than at first appears, owing to the associated movements.

Stewart (1948) states that associated movements occur more frequently after an infantile hemiplegia than after a hemiplegia in later life. Our findings suggest that they were weak in young childhood and tended to become more marked by the age of 8 or 9 years. Very few hemiplegics showed none. There seems to be some evidence that the child can learn to control these movements. Typically, a hemiplegic child runs with the upper limb in the flexed hemiplegic position, an associated movement ; but some children in our series by frequent practice can run with the arm down.

In a certain number of cases the defect was predominantly muscular, and the spasticity severe. In this type contractures were very liable to occur.

However, it was felt that at least four other types of hemiplegia were seen :—

1. Four cases showed hemiathetosis, two following birth difficulty. There were typical athetoid movements on one side only. In these cases the girth of the affected limb may be increased.

2. Another group of cases showed marked sensory loss, with spasticity present often to a minimal extent. The sensory loss took the form of an astereognosis. In some cases there was a loss of sense of position and in a very few cases a more severe loss, involving touch, pain, and temperature. The disorder of motility in some of these cases might be an apraxia and not a true spasticity.

3. In a third group, the spasticity was minimal, there was no evidence of astereognosis, and yet the child refused to use his affected arm. He would attempt very awkwardly to button his clothes with his non-affected hand, making no attempt to help with his affected hand, yet there appeared to be no obvious reason why he should not use it. It appeared as if the child had a defective body-image and forgot about his affected hand. Two rather more spastic children carried their affected arm held out behind them, and seemed unconscious of its presence unless reminded. In each case there was no sensory loss.

4. Fourthly, there was a group with minimal spasticity and often no sensory loss, but a pronounced defect in growth. Penfield and Robertson (1943) have commented on similar non-spastic cases and shown that the defect in growth could not be attributed to disuse or vasomotor disturbance, and was presumably due to definite cerebral damage. Following operation in such cases for epileptiform disturbances, the lesion was found to be in the post-central cortex.

Apart from this subdivision of hemiplegic cases, on the grounds of movement defect, these cases are also sharply divided by initial causation. About two-thirds of the cases of infantile hemiplegia appear to date from birth and have been considered developmental or congenital in origin. A third of the cases followed a known illness or catastrophe in later infancy, usually in the second year. Taylor (1952), Stewart (1948), Wyllie (1948), McGovern and Yannet (1947) in recent papers have made the clear distinction between the two types. In our series there were 69 of the first type and 28 of the second.

A possible source of error may occur in deciding into which type a case of hemiplegia falls. The movement defect in infantile hemiplegia is sometimes not apparent, even to expert

eyes, until the age of 6–8 months. As stated by Wyllie, " most
of the activities of the newborn infant depend on reflex path-
ways in the brain-stem and spinal cords and signs of pyramidal
involvement of a higher level take a variable time to appear ".
Thus in a few cases where the hemiplegia was said to have
followed an illness or catastrophe at 5–6 months, one cannot
be certain whether an hemiplegia would not have developed
in the absence of the catastrophe.

The numerical findings of the 97 cases are given below and
are subdivided into the two headings for comparison.

CONGENITAL CASES (69 *cases*)   POSTNATAL CASES (28 *cases*)

Family History.—
    7 (2 epilepsy ; 1 congenital hemi-   2 (1 cousin congenital hemiplegia ;
    plegia ; 1 (2 siblings) E.S.N. ;   1 father epilepsy).
    1 abnormal sibling ; 1 abnormal
    relative ; 1 cousin acquired
    hemiplegia).

Mother's Age at Birth.—
    Under 20 years, 0 ; 20–30 years,   Under 20 years, 1 ; 20–30 years, 12 ;
    45 ; 30–40 years, 15 ; 40+   30–40, 11 ; 40+ years, 2 ;
    years, 2 ; uncertain, 7.   uncertain, 1.

Order of Pregnancy.—
    First, 37 ; second, 16 ; third, 9 ;   First, 10 ; second, 9 ; third, 3 ;
    fourth, 5 ; uncertain, 2.   fourth+, 6.

Gestation Period.—
    Under 33 weeks, 3 ; 33–38 weeks,   Under 33 weeks, 0 ; 33–38 weeks,
    11 ; 39–42 weeks, 50 ; 43+   5 ; 39–42 weeks, 21 ; 43+
    weeks, 3 ; uncertain, 2.   weeks, 2.

Birth Process.—
    Pre-eclampsia, 15.   1.
    Other A.N. abnormality : illness,   0.
    5 ; accident, 1 ; A.P.H., 4.
    Induction, 9.   3.
    Breech, 8.   1.
    Forceps, 16.   1.
    Cæsarean, 3.   0.
    Multiple, 5.   2.
    Precipitate, 6.   3.
    Long labour, 18.   3.
    Normal full-time birth, 18.   17.
      a. With neonatal difficulty, 10.
      b. Without neonatal difficulty,
      8.
    Unknown history, 1.

Males to Females : 37 : 32.   13 : 15.

Birth Weights.—
    Under 4 lb., 5 ; 4 lb.+, 1 ; 5 lb.   Under 4 lb., 1 ; 4 lb.+, 0 ; 5 lb.+,
    +, 9 ; 6 lb.+, 14 ; 7 lb.+,   3 ; 6 lb.+, 11 ; 7 lb.+, 5 ; 8 lb.
    21 ; 8 lb.+, 11 ; 9 lb.+, 4 ;   +, 5 ; 9 lb.+, 2 ; uncertain, 1 ;
    uncertain, 3 ; premature, 14.   premature, 2.

CONGENITAL CASES (*cont.*)	POSTNATAL CASES (*cont.*)
Congenital Defects.—	
4 (1 absent corpus callosum; 1 Sterge-Weber's syndrome; 1 paralysis of eyelid; 1 blind microcephalic).	1 (Fallot's tetralogy).
Right : Left hemiplegia.—36 : 33.	
14 : 14.	
Neonatal Abnormalities.—	
Asphyxia, 25 ; uncertain, 9.	1.
Jaundice, 4.	0.
Cerebral irritation, 16.	2.
Other difficulties (feeding difficulty or very sleepy), 22.	5 (feeding difficulties).
Examination.—	
Convulsions after 4 weeks, 23.	17 (apart from original illness).
Cerebral infection or catastrophe, 0.	26.
Large head, 2.	2.
Small head, 13.	5.
Eyes.—	
Blind, 2 ; impaired, 8.	0 ; 4.
Field defect, 5.	5.
Strabismus, 11.	5.
Sensory Defects.—20.	12.
Hearing Defect.—0.	3.
Speech Defect.—12.	8.
School.—	
Ordinary school, 44.	13.
Spastic school, 1.	2.
P.H. school, 1.	2.
E.S.N., 7.	4.
Oc.C., 5.	1.
Not yet placed, 11.	6.

The 69 congenital cases will be discussed first.

FAMILY HISTORY

The family history of neurological abnormality in these cases does not appear to be significant except possibly in the third case, mentioned under ' congenital defects '. There was an incidence of two brothers with congenital left hemiplegia in one family. In both cases there was severe pre-eclampsia, followed by a difficult birth, and it is possible that the family history was a coincidence.

CASES DUE TO CONGENITAL DEFECT

Three cases were due to a congenital defect. In one case, an air encephalogram showed an absent corpus callosum. In this normally intelligent little girl, with a right hemiplegia, there was a marked variation in the movement pattern. She gave a unilateral response to normal bilateral movements. She shrugged only one shoulder and smiled with one side of her face. She had a marked astereognosis.

Another case was an example of Sturge Weber syndrome with a facial nævus, and evidence of intracranial calcification.

A third case was a blind microcephalic idiot with left hemiplegia, possibly due to congenital cerebral hemiatrophy. There was a family history of a congenital neurological abnormality in several members.

ABNORMALITY OF BIRTH PROCESS

In this group, as in other types of movement defect due to a cerebral cause, there is overriding evidence of abnormality in the birth process.

Antenatal Abnormality.—The evidence of antenatal abnormality was not pronounced. In one case of twins, the mother miscarried a triplet at 3 months, and the twins were very premature. In 2 cases of antepartum hæmorrhage, the resultant births were premature, one complicated by pre-eclampsia. In 4 cases the mother had an illness—asthma, influenza, pertussis, and an operation—which did not appear significant. One mother had rheumatic heart disease followed by a premature birth.

Pre-eclampsia.—There was a high incidence of pre-eclampsia—15 cases, and these pregnancies ended in 2 premature births, 5 forceps deliveries, 3 breech deliveries, one Cæsarean section, and 4 normal labours, preceded by induction. Two of these gave a history of antepartum hæmorrhage.

Brash (1949) showed that there is a greater liability to asphyxia in infants born of ' toxæmia ' mothers, due to antepartum hæmorrhage and placental infarction, giving a higher incidence of neonatal œdema and a higher incidence of prematurity.

The occurrence of pre-eclampsia may thus have a direct bearing on the occurrence of hemiplegia.

Birth Process.—The incidence of abnormality in the actual birth of these 69 cases is so marked that analysis is unnecessary. In fact, in only 18 cases was there a history of normal full-time birth of 24 hours' duration or less, and in 10 of these 18 cases there was evidence of difficulties in the neonatal period, either asphyxia, neonatal œdema, cerebral irritation with twitching, sleepiness, feeding difficulties, or an illness in a previously normal newborn infant.

Asphyxia Neonatorum.—In this series of cases, asphyxia appeared to be an important factor occurring in at least 25 cases. In 9 cases the baby was premature and in 7 cases because of the feeble respiratory control he was nursed in an oxygen tent. One of these premature babies was born in a caul and respiration was not established for 20 minutes. Another had, in addition, jaundice of prematurity.

In 11 cases the asphyxia followed a complicated delivery. In 4 forceps deliveries, the birth was further complicated by being the first of twins and a face presentation ; in other cases there were a persistent posterior presentation with membranes ruptured for 36 hours beforehand, a long labour in a severe pre-eclamptic, and a long labour with a transverse lie.

Four further cases of asphyxia followed a breech delivery and 2 a Cæsarean section. One followed a long labour with much sedation. It is impossible to predict in these last 12 cases to what extent the asphyxia in the baby might have been due to the anæsthetic given to the mother. The evidence in all these cases is of long, difficult, complicated labours carried out with skilled attention. All except one were delivered in hospital. Six of these 11 cases were booked or needed hospital confinement because of pre-eclampsia and 2 because of the presence of twins.

One case of spastic hemiplegia followed a precipitate delivery in a multipara.

In 4 cases the asphyxia followed a normal birth. In one case the midwife had difficulty with the cord round the neck. One case showed the condition of Sturge-Weber disease and possibly was an example of an abnormal child responding poorly to the physiological adaptation needed after birth.

Thus asphyxia must be considered a very serious factor in the causation of congenital hemiplegia.

Neonatal Jaundice.—In contrast, jaundice does not appear to be significant in the history of spastic hemiplegia. There were 4 cases, all of physiological jaundice and not due to rhesus incompatibility. One of these was known to me at birth, and the true pathology was a subdural hæmatoma (*Case* 12). One case followed a long labour with asphyxia and one a precipitate delivery. In the fourth case the full birth history could not be obtained as the parents were abroad. The few cases of neonatal jaundice in this series is in marked contrast to the athetoid group of cases and differs considerably from the incidence in paraplegias and quadriplegias.

Caput Succedaneum.—In 4 cases there was a history of marked cranial moulding after birth, in 3 following a normal birth and in one following a long labour. Byers (1941) has suggested that caput succedaneum can cause underlying cerebral œdema and venous engorgement and hæmorrhage leading to hemiplegia. In one case it was possible to confirm that the encephalohæmatoma—an allied condition—was on the suspected side. In all 4 cases the hemiplegia was minimal. This may be a significant finding.

Neonatal Illness.—Following this history of abnormal birth, there was symptomatic evidence of cerebral damage in 32 cases. This took the form of cerebral irritations and twitching, excessive sleepiness with inability to rouse, and sucking difficulties.

In 6 cases the child appeared normal at birth and gave no worry for several days after until it suddenly collapsed and was obviously ill. In 2 of these cases a subdural hæmatoma was diagnosed and treated. There must have been underlying cerebral damage, as it is known that subdural hæmatoma can be treated at birth with no sequelæ. Presumably a meningeal hæmorrhage as described by Sarah McNutt in 1885 had taken place.

Three case histories are given and show that although the child's condition at birth was apparently normal cerebral damage had occurred.

Case 11.—The fourth child, born at home after a normal delivery, weighing 7 lb. At 3 days of age she was admitted urgently to hospital with signs of cerebral irritation and bulging fontanelle. An encephalo-hæmatoma was present. A right subdural hæmatoma was found and the child was treated surgically. Subsequently a hydrocephalus developed, presumably due to defective absorption from the damaged arachnoid membrane. The child suffered from fits from 2 months of age. She was later found to have a severe left hemiplegia and the spasm of the trunk muscles had caused a subluxation of the left hip. She was blind and an imbecile.

Case 12.—The second child, born after a normal delivery, weighing 6 lb. 8 oz. There was a family history of fits. At 8 days of age she became ill and excessively flaccid, refusing her feeds. A right subdural hæmatoma was discovered and treated. She was later found to have a left spastic hemiplegia which responded well to treatment. In addition, her right arm was found to be flaccid and shorter than the left. Whether this was due to an Erb's palsy or to cerebral damage of area 6 was not decided. Her intelligence was normal, she walked at 3 years, and later attended ordinary school.

A different pathology may have accounted for one other case showing sudden neonatal illness.

Case 13.—The fourth child, born after a forceps delivery complicated by slight pre-eclampsia, weighing 8 lb. 6 oz. He appeared well at birth, but at the age of 5 days became ill and comatosed with marked œdema. His weight went down to 6 lb. He later developed into a boy of normal intelligence with a severe right spastic hemiplegia. There was a field of vision defect and a marked sensory loss both of astereognosis and sense of position. He had his first fit at 9 years of age and an air encephalogram revealed cerebral atrophy at that time. Subsequently the fits became more severe and prevented him from obtaining employment. He was treated by parieto-occipital lobectomy in April, 1954, with marked success. He now has a permanent clerical job. The removed portion of brain showed the walnut appearance of several fibrosed gyra in the parieto-occipital area, presumably due to venous damage at birth.

Possibly the other 3 cases giving a history of normal birth were of this type and similar to the cases where brain damage had been suspected from birth.

From all these facts the evidence of cerebral damage during the birth process was very strong. On the other hand a careful analysis of all the findings shows very little evidence of unskilled or meddlesome midwifery. The difficulties may have been unavoidable. In fact in very few cases could it be said that the mother had an imagined grievance against the obstetrician or midwife. In many cases the mothers were consciously or subconsciously blaming themselves and this feeling of guilt was a serious factor in their attitude to their handicapped child.

Out of the 69 cases, 43 were born in hospital, 12 in nursing homes, 11 at home, and in 3 the place of confinement was unknown.

CLINICAL FINDINGS

In addition to the movement defect these cases of congenital hemiplegia showed other clinical abnormalities which will be discussed in detail in later chapters. In particular there was evidence of defective vision, and defective eye movements, speech defects, a cortical sensory loss, and a high incidence of fits.

Affected Side.—Perlstein (1953) states that in congenital premature cases the incidence of right to left hemiplegia was 1 : 1. In full-time cases he states that the incidence of right to left is 2 : 1. He explains this by stating that the left occipito-anterior position of a normal delivery is more common than the right occipito-anterior position. McGovern and Yannet (1947) state that after birth trauma the incidence of right to left is 2 : 20, but that 'developmental' cases were more frequently on the right side.

Our findings do not entirely fit in with these statements. Among the 14 premature cases there were 8 right and 6 left hemiplegias. Among the rest (neglecting the 3 congenital cases which were 1 right and 2 left) the proportion was 28 : 24. Omitting the 30 cases of breech, forceps, Cæsarean cases, and congenital defects which would not necessarily be influenced by the presentation, the proportion was 20 : 19. Thus, on the evidence of these small numbers no factor could be found which influenced one side or the other.

Air Encephalogram.—An air encephalogram was obtained in 13 cases. One case revealed the interesting condition of absent corpus callosum and one confirmed the diagnosis of Sturge-Weber disease. Another was normal in a case of hemi-athetosis. The remaining 10 cases all showed dilatation of the lateral ventricle on the affected side with evidence of unilateral cerebral atrophy. In some cases there was deviation of the third ventricle to the affected side. As stated by Crothers and Wyatt (1941) this may be a favourable sign and may suggest that the non-affected hemisphere is growing normally and displacing the defective hemisphere. In one case in which the hemiplegia had followed a normal birth and neonatal period, the air encephalogram showed cerebral atrophy thus suggesting cerebral damage, although there had been no suggestive clinical history.

DISCUSSION

Following a full statement of the aetiological findings in this interesting group of 69 cases of congenital hemiplegia, one is left in some doubt as to the underlying pathology.

In the first 3 congenital cases the pathology seems certain. In the 2 cases of hemiathetosis there may have been unilateral venous damage to a branch of the vein of Galen following asphyxia, causing scarring in the corpus striatum. A condition of unilateral *état marbré* may be present similar to that occurring in the bilateral cases of athetosis mentioned later.

In the remaining cases the evidence is suggestive of cerebral atrophy on the affected side with coincidental internal hydrocephalus and enlargement of the lateral ventricle. The cerebral atrophy was presumably due to damage during the birth process or in the immediate neonatal period. It is suggested that in some cases there has been venous thrombosis or engorgement and hæmorrhage in the veins leading into the longitudinal sinus on one side, causing scarring, ulegyria, and cerebral atrophy with compensatory enlargement of the lateral ventricle. The area of damage may be precentral involving the motor areas or postcentral involving the sensory areas. In other cases there may be more pronounced involvement of the parietal or occipital lobes and in a few cases the temporal lobes. In cases of field of vision defect, mentioned later, there must have been involvement of the occipital areas or the optic radiations in the depths of the parietal areas. The evidence is in favour of a catastrophe of vascular origin or an anoxia causing damage to one hemisphere only.

It has been suggested by Wyllie (1948) and Carmichael (1954) that in some cases the condition may be due to an embolus in a branch of the middle cerebral artery and it has been suggested that this embolus might be a placental villus. This catastrophe may have occurred in some of the serious cases, but it seems more likely in the mild cases that the damage was venous in origin. This pathology was suggested in the one case of hemispherectomy.

A cause of congenital hemiplegia mentioned by Ford (1944) is a condition of cerebral hemiatrophy, with the two hemispheres unequally developed, and the cortical pattern on the affected side being normal or of primitive type. It seems difficult to decide whether any of the cases in this survey could be of this pattern. As the majority show evidence of birth trauma, it seems unlikely, except in the one case already mentioned.

POSTNATAL HEMIPLEGIA

Under this heading are included all the cases—28 in number —in which the hemiplegia developed in later childhood after a known illness or catastrophe. In some cases the onset of the illness was very sudden with convulsions and coma in a previously healthy child. In other cases the hemiplegia was first noted during the course of a known infectious illness or septic condition. Occasionally hemiplegia follows cerebral trauma. In two of our cases it was insidious in onset.

As stated by Wyllie (1948), "this term [infantile hemiplegia] has been in use since the middle of the nineteenth century to denote certain cases of hemiplegia of sudden tempestuous onset in children of a few weeks to 6 or more years of age ".

As also noted by Wyllie in a number of cases there was a prior history of a difficult birth with neonatal symptoms. This had occurred in 7 of our cases and in 4 there was some doubt as to whether the child was normal before the catastrophe which led to the hemiplegia. It is suggested by Wyllie " that confluent petechial hæmorrhages or necrotic areas due to asphyxial venous congestion at birth may coalesce and lead to a large trabeculated cystic cavity in the white matter of one hemisphere ". Norman (1947) suggests that the " original lesions spare sufficient cortical tissues to mask for the time being the inherent instability of the infant's motor apparatus. But as sclerosis gradually increases, epileptogenic foci are formed, convulsions begin and hemiplegia is precipitated."

The numerical findings have been given in comparison with cases of congenital hemiplegia. There appear to be various childhood illnesses which may lead to hemiplegia. As they represent a wide variety of clinical conditions the cases are described in some detail with a number of medical histories.

GROUP 1. HEMIPLEGIA FOLLOWING SUDDEN ILLNESS

The condition of hemiplegia may follow a sudden unexplained illness in a previously normal child. This was apparently noted by Hippocrates, who mentions in his writings that hemiplegia may follow a fit. Taylor in 1905 described the condition : " a child hitherto healthy suddenly becomes ill without any apparent cause between the age of 1 month and 6 years. The early symptoms are severe and consist of convulsions, fever, often vomiting, always coma."

A sudden illness of this type occurred in 11 of our cases, but in 5 of them there was evidence of developmental abnormality before the illness. The pathology in these 5 cases presumably follows the pattern suggested by Norman. In 3 of these cases the hemiplegia did not follow the first, but a subsequent fit.

Case 14.—A second child, born after two inductions and an undiagnosed twin pregnancy, at 37 weeks. She was the second twin and weighed 5 lb. 8 oz. and suffered from blue asphyxia at birth. She was an abnormal child from birth. A right internal strabismus was noted immediately and she was late in reaching her milestones. She suffered from mild fits. At 2 years 2 months she was admitted to an Isolation Hospital with a mild attack of pertussis and after a fit the spastic hemiplegia was noted. She continued to have fits. There was impaired vision due to a cortical cause with slight nystagmus. Her I.Q. was 60. The E.E.G. showed the left hemisphere to be completely silent with ' bursts ' from the right side. The A.E.G. showed left-sided cerebral atrophy.

In the other 6 cases there was every evidence of a healthy child before the illness.

Case 15.—A second child, born after a normal delivery, weighing 6 lb. 15 oz. at birth. He appeared well until 6 weeks of age when he went into a severe convulsion while being bathed. He was taken to hospital and intracranial hæmorrhage was diagnosed. Subsequently he was found to have a right hemiplegia with marked wasting. There was astereognosis and a doubtful field of vision defect. He had occasional convulsions and frequent temper tantrums. He was microcephalic and had an I.Q. of 72 (his brother's I.Q. was 140).

The E.E.G. showed a lack of left-sided activity and the A.E.G. showed gross dilatation of the left lateral ventricle with little evidence of cerebral tissue on that side.

In the other 5 cases a similar story was obtained. In a child of 2 years the hemiplegia appeared to be accompanied by defective sight and hearing and a sensory aphasia, all of cerebral origin. As the child got older these faculties slowly returned and there seemed to be some evidence at $2\frac{1}{2}$ years that she was beginning to understand.

From the hospital notes a similar story seemed to have occurred in a girl now aged 13 years. Her sight, hearing, and understanding had been very defective immediately after the illness. At the age of 13 years she was an educationally subnormal girl, who still had some evidence of motor aphasia. There was athetosis in the affected arm and astereognosis was also present. The E.E.G. showed a lesion in the right temporal region with a liability to fits. Petit mal attacks commenced in adolescence.

Of these 6 children, 4 are educationally subnormal, one is above normal (without fits), and one not yet determined ; 5 are having fits.

In cases of this type a vascular catastrophe is thought to have occurred. Vascular occlusions in the branches of the middle cerebral or anterior cerebral arteries have been reported at post-mortem by Wyllie (1948), Ford and Schaffer (1927), and in cases following hemispherectomy (Carmichael, 1954). Some cases may be due to venous occlusion. The theory of Strumpell (1884) that there may be cases of polio-encephalitis is not now accepted.

GROUP 2. HEMIPLEGIA FOLLOWING AN INFECTIOUS FEVER

Infectious fever is another known cause of hemiplegia and 2 cases occurred in this series, one following chicken-pox and the other pertussis.

Case 16.—The third child born after a normal delivery, weighing 8 lb. 12 oz. at birth. At the age of 9 months he was taken suddenly ill with severe fits and the rash of chicken-pox developed a few hours later. On recovery a right hemiplegia was noted. From that time he had occasional epileptic and petit mal attacks. His behaviour was uncontrolled. At the age of 9 years his I.Q. was 74, and the E.E.G. showed focal disturbance in the right temporal region. The A.E.G. showed dilatation of the left lateral ventricle with displacement of the ventricular system to that side. The possible pathology in this case may be an acute encephalomyelitis due to the virus infection, or a vascular catastrophe due to toxic damage to a vessel-wall. More likely, as suggested by Wyllie (1948), it was an allergic condition, a specific brain antibody-antigen reaction, leading to a cortical demyelinization as suggested later.

In the following case of post-pertussis hemiplegia there remains the possibility that the true pathology is venous damage during a severe coughing spasm.

Case 17.—A second child, born after a precipitate delivery, weighing 8 lb. 10 oz. At 27 months of age she had a particularly severe attack of pertussis and during its course she was taken suddenly ill with convulsions. A right spastic hemiplegia was noted afterwards.

At 5 years of age she was found to have a slight right hemiplegia with no wasting or shortening. She had had very adequate physiotherapy treatment and could dorsiflex her foot well. There was a doubtful loss of sense of position and astereognosis on the affected side. She had occasional fits and was distractible and restless. Her face was rather more affected than is usual. Her I.Q. was 98 and the E.E.G. showed a disturbance from the left central area.

GROUP 3. POST-IMMUNIZATION HEMIPLEGIA

Following this account of 2 cases precipitated by an infectious fever, there were 2 cases which appeared to follow immunization or vaccination. It is suggested in these cases that the pathology may be one of allergy with œdema and extravasation around cerebral capillaries, causing necrosis of brain-cells and eventual demyelinization, as is suggested in the cases of infectious fever.

Case 18.—The second child, born after a normal delivery, weighing 5 lb. 8 oz. She was a healthy little girl, walking and talking, when at 18 months of age she had a fit lasting half-an-hour preceding an attack of German measles. She was immunized against diphtheria and pertussis four months later and was " quite ill " after the first injection. Thirteen days after the second injection she had an attack of severe convulsions which lasted four hours. She was unconscious for three days afterwards and on recovery was noted to have a flaccid paralysis of the right arm and leg. She appeared to be blind and deaf. There were nystagmoid movements to the right. Over a period of weeks her condition gradually improved and the flaccid paralysis gave place to a right spastic paralysis. Her hearing and sight gradually returned and were eventually thought to be normal. For months she did not appear to understand and she had no speech. Gradually these two faculties returned and by the age of 3½ years she had begun to talk. There appeared to be no field of vision defect. Sensation and intelligence could not be tested. She suffered from slight epileptiform attacks which were controlled with drugs. At 5 years she was found to be educationally subnormal.

Case 19.—A first child, born after a normal delivery, weighing 9 lb. 2 oz. He was vaccinated at 6 weeks of age. At 3 months of age he had an illness which was diagnosed as vaccinal encephalitis with convulsive movements down the left side. A left spastic hemiplegia was noted afterwards. At 9 years of age the spasticity was slight but there was ½ in. shortening of the upper limb and ¾ in. shortening of the lower limb. There was a sensory loss to superficial sensation, sense of position, and an astereognosis. He had no sense of position in his toes and was liable to crowd them into his shoes with toes flexed, causing a blister (*Fig.* 11). His mother had to make sure his toes were properly placed in his shoes and, for instance, put on his football boots for him before he went to school. He had no field of vision defect. His I.Q. was 106 and he was making good educational progress. Whether the diagnosis was vaccinal encephalitis remains in doubt. There may have been a vascular catastrophe.

The neurological sequelæ of prophylactic inoculation was the subject of an article by Miller and Stanton (1954), and in their series hemiplegia occurred after whooping-cough immunization.

GROUP 4. HEMIPLEGIA FOLLOWING AN INFECTIVE CONDITION

This condition may occur both in children and adults and the possible cause in the following 2 cases is cortical damage from a venous thrombosis.

Case 20.—A second child, born after a normal delivery, weighing 7 lb. 12 oz. At 2 years 10 months he was treated surgically for a gangrenous appendix with pelvic abscess. He made a slow recovery and a right spastic hemiplegia was first noted by his mother as soon as he returned home. The condition appeared to be chiefly a muscular defect. There was no sensory loss, defect in growth, or field of vision defect, or aphasia. The boy was unusual in that he held his affected hand in exactly the opposite way to a normal hemiplegic. The upper limb was held abducted, externally rotated with elbow extension and supination and finger and wrist hyperextended. He walked with his hand away from and behind him as if unconscious of it. He may have had some loss of body-image. Later, he improved considerably and began to use his arm quite well although it remained

4

stiff. The A.E.G. and E.E.G. at age 3½ years were normal and his I.Q. was 100.

Case 21.—A fourth child, born after a normal delivery, weighing 7 lb. 8 oz. He had an empyema at 11 months and the condition of left spastic hemiplegia was noted in hospital during the illness. In this case the hemiplegia was particularly severe. There were marked contraction deformities with shortening of the arm. It was difficult to be certain about sensory loss as the use of the hand was so poor. His I.Q. was 69. There was no visual field defect. He suffered from fits of a petit mal type. An A.E.G. showed " dilatation of the left lateral ventricle without displacement consistent with some degree of cerebral atrophy ". This interesting A.E.G. suggested that the cerebral atrophy was on the same side as the hemiplegia. The possible explanation is that there was mild damage on the right side giving the left hemiplegia, and more severe cortical atrophy on the left, possibly a factor in the low mentality (*Fig.* 12).

In 2 cases the condition followed a known attack of meningo-coccal meningitis. In these cases the residual defect was mild and the intelligence good. Again the suggestive pathology is a venous thrombosis following the infective condition.

Another case followed a cerebral abscess at the age of 8 months. This child with a right hemiplegia had a low intelligence and frequent epileptiform attacks resembling petit mal. There was evidence of residual motor aphasia.

A further case with a history of pneumonia was interesting because of the evidence of widespread cerebral damage co-existent with a superior intelligence.

Case 22.—The first of twins born after a first pregnancy to a mother of 39 years. The boy weighed 3 lb. 8 oz. at birth and gave some neonatal worry and had feeding difficulties. He developed normally until 5 years of age, when he had a fall and was unconscious for a short period. Pneumonia followed and the right hemiplegia was noted afterwards. When seen at the age of 13 years 10 months he had a mild right spastic hemiplegia with ½ in. shortening of upper and lower limbs. There was a defective temperature apprecia-tion, a loss of sense of position and vibration, and astereognosis. He had a field of vision defect of which he became aware only after the examination. He had an internal strabismus of the right eye. His head circumference was 19½ in. There had been no fits. His I.Q. was 132. He was neat, precise, enjoyed mental exertion, and was doing well at a Grammar School. He was left-eyed. Apart from the neurological findings, the size of the head suggested severe brain damage. The original cause of the condition, whether due to birth damage, trauma at 5 years, or pneumonia, remains obscure.

GROUP 5. HEMIPLEGIA FOLLOWING TUBERCULOSIS

There were 2 cases of hemiplegia following tuberculosis. One child had had tuberculous meningitis at 10 months and the condition of left hemiplegia was noted after some months of treatment. The hemiplegia was athetoid in character in both arm and leg (*Fig.* 13). She carried her hand behind her and seemed to have some loss of sense of body-image. There was no sensory loss or field of vision defect. The E.E.G. was highly abnormal, suggesting involvement of deep and superficial structures to right of midline with a liability to cerebral instability. Her I.Q. was 66.

The other case—a left hemiplegia—followed an operation for tuberculous mesenteric adenitis with abscess in the hypochondrium at 3 years of age. A radiograph taken several years later showed three calcified foci in the right parietal region and an A.E.G. showed a porencephaly communicating with the right lateral ventricle. This condition was presumably associated with the original tuberculous illness.

GROUP 6. HEMIPLEGIA FOLLOWING SYPHILIS

One case of left hemiplegia followed a fit at 13 months in a child already considered abnormal. Congenital syphilis was present and may have been the deciding factor.

GROUP 7. HEMIPLEGIA FOLLOWING TRAUMA

One case followed a fall on the head at 5 months of age, with a period of unconsciousness. The skull was not fractured.

GROUP 8. HEMIPLEGIA FOLLOWING CONGENITAL HEART DISEASE

A right hemiplegia developed at the age of 1 year in a boy suffering from Fallot's tetralogy. He had a sensory loss, and a good intelligence. (*Fig.* 14.) Ford (1944) suggests that these cases are due to cerebral thrombosis.

GROUP 9. HEMIPLEGIA OF INSIDIOUS ONSET

Lastly, 2 cases came on insidiously, both in children of 11 years.

Case 23.—A first child, born after a medical and surgical induction for small maternal measurements. The gestation period was 37 weeks and she weighed 5 lb. 3 oz. at birth. There were no neonatal worries.

She suffered from infantile eczema and asthma. A left hemiplegia developed gradually at 11 years with no history of illness. When she was first seen by the team at 13 years of age the history suggested that the condition was considerably more advanced than it had been two years previously. The spasticity was marked, with shortening and wasting in upper and lower limb. There were defective sense of position in arm and leg and astereognosis in the arm. She had a visual field defect. Her I.Q. was 80, but her vocabulary level was above her intelligence level, suggesting intellectual deterioration. There had been no fits. The A.E.G. showed marked cortical atrophy.

Here again the cause is in doubt. Following the premature birth, there may have been brain damage with insidious sclerosis which eventually revealed itself as a hemiplegia. Alternatively, the pathology may be one of cortical demyelinization following the allergic condition of eczema and asthma.

The other child was said to have deteriorated following an attack of pertussis with convulsions at 4 years. She was always backward, and the hemiplegia developed insidiously at 11 years with occasional fits.

DISCUSSION

These 28 cases all living in the Bristol Clinical Area represent a medley of clinical conditions of widely differing aetiology, whose end-result produced a similar movement-pattern defect.

After the serious illness precipitating the hemiplegia, the total cerebral disorientation of the child appears to be marked (as mentioned by Asher and Schonell, 1950). There was a sensory loss in at least 12 cases, a field of vision defect in 5, and impaired vision in 4. There was evidence of an aphasia in 3, and in 9 there was a speech defect, considered to be due to mental backwardness in 7.

Following the original convulsive illness, fits continued to occur in 18 out of the 28 cases, and E.E.G. findings suggest the possibility of future fits in 2 more. The cerebral disturbance has severely upset the behaviour of these children and in at least 10 cases the children were distractible and hyperexcitable. They were difficult to manage and educate and possibly the cerebral instability will cause concern in later years.

There was also evidence of a loss of general intelligence. The I.Q. levels obtained were :—

Range	Number
Under 50	4
50–69	7
70–89	6
90–109	6
110–129	1
130	1

Three cases were still recovering from the illness and were untestable.

SUMMARY

Ninety-seven cases of hemiplegia are discussed.

The movement defect is described in detail.

Four variations in the type of defect are described :—

a. There may be a hemiathetosis.

b. The poverty of movement may be due to a cortical sensory loss.

c. Bizarre movements may be due to a loss of body-image.

d. Defect in growth may be the overriding handicap.

Sixty-nine cases appeared to be congenital in origin. Of these, 3 were due to a congenital abnormality.

The remaining 66 cases showed a high incidence of an abnormal birth, neonatal asphyxia, and neonatal illness.

There appeared to be no factor which influenced the development of the hemiplegia on one side of the body in preference to the other.

Twenty-eight cases followed an illness in later infancy.

These cases and the probable causes are described in detail.

The total cerebral disorientation following this infantile illness appeared to be profound.

CHAPTER VIII

QUADRIPLEGIA

In this group of severely handicapped children spasticity involves all four limbs, and it is to this type of case that the term ' Little's Disease ' is usually applied. Here again the pattern of movement defect is not uniform and various types are seen and are illustrated in *Figs.* 15–22.

In some cases of quadriplegia the legs are affected more than the arms and the condition in the legs is approximately symmetrical and similar to that seen in the severest type of paraplegia. Some of these cases appear to follow a premature birth. In full extension, either supine or erect, there is adduction and internal rotation of the hips, extension at the knees, and extreme plantar flexion at the feet, giving the picture of 'scissors gait'. Coupled with the extreme spasticity of the lower limbs, the upper limbs may be very mildly, mildly, or severely affected. In the very mild cases there may be a retraction of the shoulders with pectoral spasm and often a tendency to kyphosis and an impression that the hands are stiff and awkwardly used. In mild cases there is definite spasticity around the elbow joints with a difficulty to supinate, and a more marked stiffness and uselessness of the hands. In the severe cases, the whole upper limb is held in the typical spastic pattern with flexion, adduction, and internal rotation of the shoulders, flexion of the elbows, pronation of the forearm, and flexion of the wrist and finger-joints with inversion of the thumb so that it is pressed into the palm by the flexion of the fingers. In some postures the head is hyperextended, in which case the arms are abducted and externally rotated at the shoulders with flexion of the elbows. There is often also a bilateral internal strabismus of the eyes.

In all these grades of spastic quadriplegia there is some evidence of symmetry. The condition of the lower limbs is

similar.   However, because a child of even poor intelligence
will make some effort to use his hands, it is usually found that
the dominant arm is very much better than the other which is,
perhaps, an indication of the improvement that can be obtained
with treatment.   Some cases that may truly have been symmetrical quadriplegics with legs worse than arms, appear in
later childhood to be cases of triplegia with one arm nearly
normal, because of the marked improvement.   Usually the
parents, and in some cases the child himself, will remember that
one arm was ' bad '.   I have personally, over a period of years,
seen cases of quadriplegia appear to turn into triplegia.   This
may have been a factor complicating other figures of symmetrical and asymmetrical quadriplegia.   It is suggested that
the term 'symmetrical quadriplegia' should be confined to cases
where the movement defect in the legs is of approximately
equal severity.

In a second rather different type of quadriplegia the condition
of the arms is worse than the legs and usually the whole of
one side is more affected than the other.   These cases have
been called asymmetrical quadriplegias and some may be
bilateral hemiplegias.   Here again, one arm may be much
improved with use, and the condition of the legs may have
remained static due to the inability to walk, and again, in these
cases, it cannot be said that both arms are worse than the legs.
The asymmetrical cases appear to follow birth trauma rather
than prematurity, and the diagnosis of bilateral hemiplegia
is suggested by the fact that in one or two more intelligent
cases a bilateral astereognosis has been found.

Other slightly rarer and more bizarre combinations of
spastic quadriplegia and triplegia may be seen.   Occasionally
one arm and the alternate leg are worse affected.   In other cases
there seems to be evidence of a hemiplegia on one side with
a general awkwardness of movement on the other side.   The
possibility of a bilateral abnormality may also be suggested by
a definite motor speech defect.   On some occasions it has
been thought possible that on the less affected side we are
dealing with a condition which in adults would be called
apraxia.   In fact, Brain (1955) has suggested that an extensive
lesion in one hemisphere can cause a contralateral hemiplegia

and an ipsolateral apraxia due to both precentral area and parietal lobe damage. It is purely conjectural as to whether we are occasionally meeting this abnormality in children.

It is possible to meet a condition of athetosis in the arms and spasticity in the legs. This condition has been met in premature children, and may be a combination of the typical symmetrical spastic paraplegia with additional damage to the basal ganglia leading to athetosis.

The term diplegia has been applied variously by writers to all types of quadriplegia and is therefore not used in this survey.

In some ways the movement upset in quadriplegics is similar to that described later in athetosis. There is a disturbance in the normal appearance or disappearance of infantile reflexes. There is often evidence of the presence of an asymmetric tonic neck reflex, even in a mild case (*Fig.* 17 B). On turning the head, the ' skull ' arm flexes and the ' jaw ' arm extends and the alternate leg extends or flexes. Also, the strong persistence of symmetrical tonic neck reflexes upsets the development of normal movement pattern. If the child is held prone with the head flexed and in the midline, the arms are abducted, externally rotated, and flexed at the elbows, the child cannot bring them forward to crawl (*Fig.* 19). The child may be able to put one arm down and not the other. On the other hand, owing to the persistence of symmetrical tonic neck reflexes, if the head is held extended in the midline the child can bring his arm down on the ground ready for crawling, but there is reflex flexor movement of the legs which prevents crawling even in this position. When the head is flexed, the elbows are flexed, and the legs severely extended at hips, knees, and ankles. When the head is extended, the arms are extended, but the lower limbs are then severely flexed at hip, knees, and ankle. There is also an absence of the power of reciprocation, which is present in a normal baby of 5 months, both lower limbs tending to move as a whole in flexion or extension. When these children begin to crawl, they tend to ' bunny hop ' with both limbs alternately flexed and extended, and are unable to carry out a normal crawl with alternate movements of arms and legs.

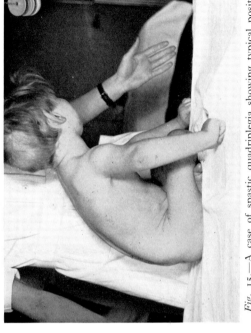

Fig. 15.—A case of spastic quadriplegia showing typical position in flexion.

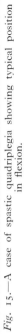

Fig. 16.—A case of spastic quadriplegia showing typical position in extension.

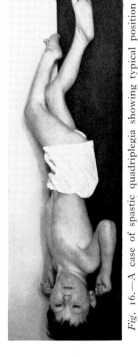

Fig. 14.—A case of right hemiplegia which developed at one year of age and was associated with Fallot's tetralogy. Marked astereognosis. Normal intelligence.

PLATE VII

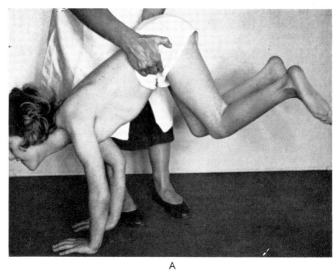

A

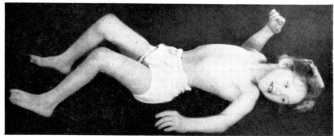

B

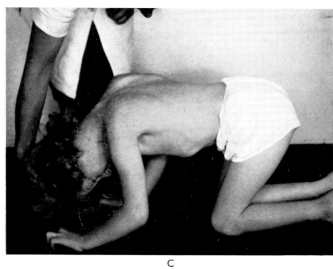

C

PLATE VIII

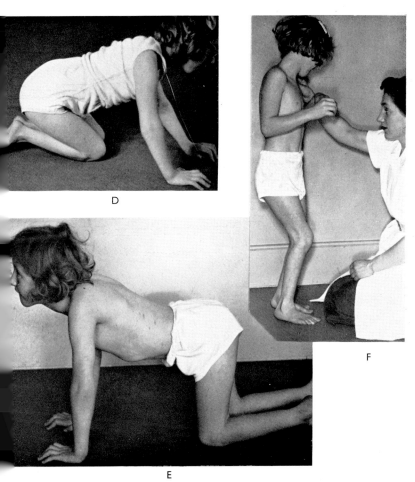

Fig. 17.—A case of spastic quadriplegia (birth weight 1 lb. 15 oz.)
showing **A**, Marked flexor spasm in legs ; **B**, Tonic neck reflex ;
C, Symmetrical tonic neck reflex with flexion of head and partial
extension of hips and lower extremities, and flexion of upper limb ;
D, Symmetrical tonic neck reflex with extension of head and flexion
of hips and lower extremities ; **E**, Improvement with treatment ; and
F, Early standing position after prolonged treatment.

PLATE IX

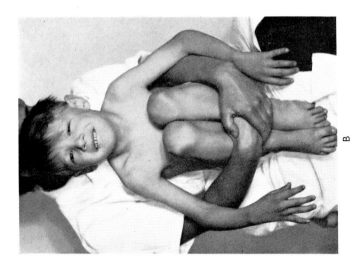

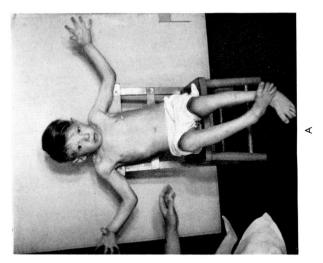

A

B

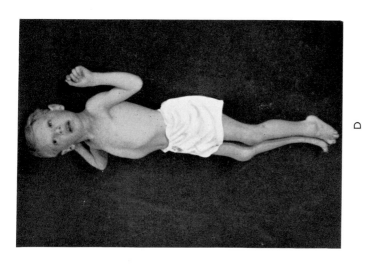

C

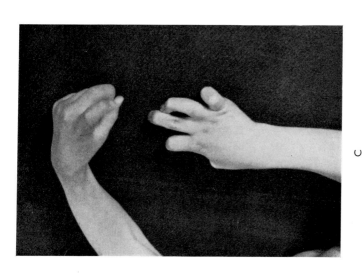

D

Fig. 18.—A case of spastic quadriplegia, possibly bilateral hemiplegia. A, Sitting posture with a tendency to extension ;
B, Sitting posture in full flexion ; C, Unusual posture of fingers ; D, Typical posture when lying supine.

PLATE XI

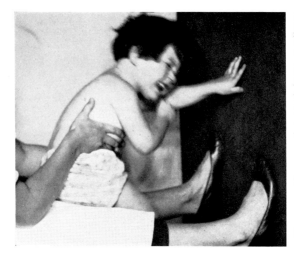

Fig. 20.—Absence of normal jump readiness due to spasticity of one arm in a case of spastic quadriplegia.

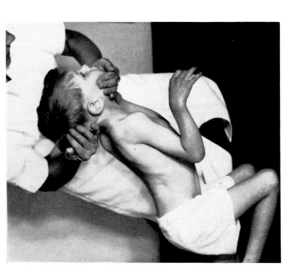

Fig. 19.—A case of spastic quadriplegia showing inability to extend arms for a normal crawl.

PLATE XII

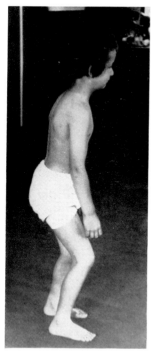

Fig. 21.—A case of triplegia showing tendency to general flexion.

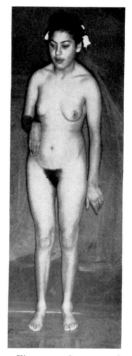

Fig. 22.—A case of spastic quadriplegia with mental deficiency which responded well to treatment and appears to be triplegic.

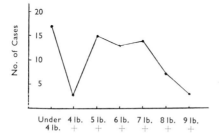

Fig. 23.—Frequency distribution of birth-weights of 72 spastic quadriplegics.

Whatever the explanation of these odd movement patterns, the muscular defect in a spastic quadriplegia can never be considered a static one, and unless the child is examined thoroughly in movement an entirely erroneous picture of the handicap may be obtained. For example, in extension either lying supine or when held erect, a spastic quadriplegic child has severe plantar flexion of the feet and is unable to dorsiflex. It may be thought that contractures are present in the calf muscles. When the same child is rolled up in a flexed position there may be marked dorsiflexion of the feet and the child is unable to plantar-flex. In a similar way adduction of the hips may appear to be extreme in a position of extension, whilst in flexion there may be quite good abduction and the child can, for instance, then sit tailor-fashion.

Although the movement upset tends to be similar in cases of spastic quadriplegia there are many differences. Some children hold their hands severely flexed with inversion of the thumb as shown (*Fig.* 18 C). In other cases the spastic position of the hand is flexion at the wrist, hyperextension at the metacarpal and phalangeal joints, and flexion at the terminal phalangeal joints. It seems difficult to explain this odd position. It may represent a return to a mammalian pattern (*Fig.* 18 C).

In spastic quadriplegia the movement patterns are abnormal because of the presence of spasticity in certain groups of muscles which can be demonstrated by the stretch reflex. The condition of spasticity, however, is not static and is present in one group of muscles and then the other, according to the posture and movement of the child. This is to be expected, as the cause of the condition is cerebral in origin and it has been said (Hughlings Jackson, 1892) that "the cortex knows nothing of muscles, it knows only movements".

In sleep the child is completely relaxed and no spasticity is present. During the survey this finding has been confirmed by visits to children late at night, and would suggest that there are no scientific grounds for the use of night splints.

If the child is maintained in a position of severe spasm for the greater part of the day, fibrous contractures of muscles can develop and severe deformities and joint dislocations result.

However, in many cases where the spasm is severe and an impression of a contracture and fixed deformity is gained, an expert physiotherapist can overcome the spasm and show that the limb or trunk is still capable of normal alinement and normal assisted and even active movements.

The figures for quadriplegia are given below, 75 cases in all.

Family History.—
    1 phenylpyruvic ; 4 epilepsy ; 3 spastic ; 1 mongol ; 1 abnormal sibling.

Mother's Age.—
    Under 20 years, 1 ; 20–30 years, 35 ; 30–40 years, 27 ; 40+ years, 6 ; uncertain, 6.

Order of Pregnancy.—
    First, 34 ; second, 18 ; third, 12 ; fourth, 8 ; uncertain, 3.

Gestation Period.—
    Under 33 weeks, 11 ; 33–38 weeks, 12 ; 39–42 weeks, 42 ; 43+ weeks, 3 ; uncertain, 7.

Birth Process.—
    Pre-eclampsia, 8.
    Antenatal abnormality, 23.
    Hæmorrhage during pregnancy, 10.
    Breech, 3.
    Brow presentation, 1.
    Forceps, 14.
    Cæsarean, 3.
    Multiple, 6.
    Long labour, 13.
    Precipitate delivery, 9.
    Normal full-time birth, 16.

Congenital Defects.—
    3 (1 cleft palate ; 1 temporal lobe agenesis ; 1 absent corpus callosum).

Birth Weights.—
    Under 4 lb., 17 ; 4 lb.+, 3 ; 5 lb.+, 15 ; 6 lb.+, 13 ; 7 lb.+, 14 ; 8 lb.+, 7 ; 9 lb.+, 3 ; uncertain, 3 ; premature, 29.

Neonatal Abnormalities.—
    Asphyxia, 30 ; uncertain, 14 ; jaundice, 10 ; cerebral irritation, 28.

*Convulsions after 4 Weeks.—*32.

Cerebral Infection or Catastrophe (in later infancy).—6.

Visual Defect.—
    Blind, 2 ; impaired vision, 19 ; field defect, 3 ; muscular imbalance, 40.

*Hearing Defect.—*4.

*Speech Defect.—*38.

Hydrocephalus.—3.
Microcephalus.—32.
School Placement.—
    O.S., 6 ; P.H., 4 ; Spastic School, 13 ; E.S.N., 4 ; Oc.C., 15 ;
    not yet placed or at home, 29 ; uncertain, 2 ; dead, 2.

AETIOLOGICAL FACTORS

Family History.—Although it is difficult to obtain controls, there appears to be a high incidence of neurological abnormality in the immediate family of a quadriplegic.   It may be that in some cases an abnormal brain has been more liable than a normal to birth damage.   This possibility is suggested by the following case.

Case 24.—The second child, born after an apparently full-time normal delivery, and weighing 5 lb.   There was a strong family history of epilepsy in the mother and other relatives.   A few days after birth the child collapsed, became cyanotic, and was treated in an oxygen tent.   He grew up to be a blind spastic quadriplegic idiot having daily fits.   The blindness was cerebral in origin.   He died aged 6 years and the brain was obtained for examination.   There appeared to be a double pathology.   There was a temporal lobe agenesis, presumably genetic, and there were ulegyria in the parieto-occipital region suggesting corticovenous thrombosis at birth.

Congenital Defects.—In 2 cases the true cause of the spastic quadriplegia appeared to be a congenital defect.

One case which presented as a typical spastic quadriplegic was found to have phenylpyruvic oligophrenia.   There was a history of a spastic sibling, 10 years older, who was in a mental institution.   The other case was as follows.

Case 25.—A first child, born after a 4-day confinement and forceps delivery, weighing 9 lb. 6 oz. at birth.   There were neonatal cerebral symptoms and a cerebral cry.   He developed into a severe hyper-kinetic spastic imbecile.   The left leg was worse than the right.   A radiograph showed an abnormal cerebral vault with diminished A.P. dimension.   An A.E.G. showed lateral ventricles somewhat separated with the third ventricle high up between them, suggesting a defect in the corpus callosum, either genetic or traumatic.

Statistics.—As this group is larger in number it is possible to make some statistical statements.   The figures show that there is a higher than average incidence of first births, and the age of the mother at the birth of the child is slightly above normal.   On analysing the birth-weight there is a marked excess of very premature births, an excess of slightly premature births, and a slight excess of children in the higher birth-weights. These last three factors are shown in a graph (*Fig.* 23). This bimodal pattern of birth-weights has been observed by Evans and Childs (1954). In itself it suggests more than one clinical cause for the condition.

Antenatal Abnormalities.—

*Antenatal Illness.—*The occurrence of antenatal illness appears to have some bearing on the incidence of prematurity. The 2 cases of antenatal pyelitis, the 1 case of excessive vomiting necessitating hospitalization, and 3 of the cases of antepartum hæmorrhage appeared to have precipitated the premature birth.

In 4 cases it was felt that a severe antenatal illness might have been the causative factor in the child's defective cerebral development. In one case the mother had influenza when two months pregnant and became unconscious. The baby was later delivered at full-time by forceps delivery, with no neonatal symptoms, and developed into a microcephalic child with particularly severe spasticity and mental retardation. In another case a similar microcephalic, severely spastic, imbecile child with epilepsy was born after a normal birth, the only significant history being a severe attack of maternal influenza at 16 weeks. In a third case the mother suffered from an A.P.H. when two months pregnant and jaundice at 4 months. The baby was delivered by forceps at 38 weeks, and was " very ill " afterwards. She was a severe spastic quadriplegic idiot. In the fourth case the mother had a known attack of German measles at 6 weeks, and the child was born at 38 weeks, weighing 3 lb. 12 oz. He had defective sight, typical spastic quadriplegia, and was educationally subnormal with an I.Q. of 56.

The significance of the antenatal story cannot be assessed, but the extreme backwardness in these 4 cases was of a rather different pattern from some of the others. One of these children spent 2 years at a Spastic School and showed no sign of understanding what was said to him. In most cases of cerebral palsy with a suggestive history of brain damage, one gets the impression of a good brain damaged, whereas in some others the impression is of a congenital idiot. One wonders if the latter cases are due to genetic causes or to antenatal illness causing a developmental defect.

Pre-eclampsia.—Eight mothers gave a history of this condition. In 5 cases it appeared to be the cause of a premature birth. In one case the birth was induced because of pre-eclampsia and in another case there was an A.P.H. In 2 further cases the pregnancy ended with a forceps delivery, blue asphyxia in the baby, and neonatal cerebral signs. The other slight case was not significant as it was one of acquired quadriplegia at 10 months.

Thus in this group, as in the hemiplegic group, pre-eclampsia as suggested by Brash (1949) can be a factor in the history of cerebral palsy by precipitating a premature birth or an antepartum hæmorrhage, or by causing postnatal asphyxia possibly related to placental insufficiency.

Antepartum Hæmorrhage.—Apart from cases of antepartum hæmorrhage followed by a premature birth or associated with pre-eclampsia, the history of a hæmorrhage during pregnancy may of itself be an important and deleterious event. There were 4 cases with a history of uterine hæmorrhage between the second and eighth months in which the baby suffered from severe postnatal asphyxia. In only one case was the birth abnormal ; and so again there is a suggestion of placental insufficiency. Three of these 4 cases were at the idiot or imbecile level.

In 2 further cases of uterine hæmorrhage one was more truly a case of rhesus incompatibility and one was a severe case of placenta prævia treated by Willett's forceps.

Ten cases of hæmorrhage during pregnancy out of 75 cases appears to be a high figure, although it is difficult to obtain accurate figures of normal incidence. There was evidence, however, in this series that the uterine hæmorrhage, whether occurring in a normal or abnormal number of cases, was a possibly significant factor in the eventual cerebral defect. It has been suggested that after a hæmorrhage in early pregnancy placental insufficiency may be present and it is unwise to allow the pregnancy to continue over 40 weeks. In these 10 cases only one mother stated that she was overdue—3 weeks.

Antenatal Fœtal Distress.—A further antenatal factor in the causation of spastic quadriplegia was a history of fœtal distress. One mother had a normal birth at home at 43 weeks' gestation, after she had passed meconium-stained liquor for a week beforehand. The child was a spastic quadriplegic idiot. In 3 further cases there was a history of the passage of meconium-stained liquor for some hours before delivery. One of these cases was delivered by Cæsarean section for fœtal distress. In a further case the membranes ruptured 4 days before birth and there was a difficult forceps delivery. All these 5 cases suffered from asphyxia and neonatal cerebral irritation. In one case xanthocromic fluid was found in the C.S.F. ; presumably there had been either a cerebral damage or an asphyxial venous engorgement with extravasation.

Birth Process.—

Prematurity.—No fewer than 29 of these 75 cases were premature and 17 were under 4 lb. at birth. These 29 cases can be further analysed and the true clinical condition elucidated.

One had evidence of rhesus incompatibility which was presumably the cause of the cerebral pathology. One weighing 5 lb. 8 oz. was *Case* 31 with acquired quadriplegia (*see later*). Two cases weighing 5 lb. 8 oz. appear to be more truly cases that come under the heading of an abnormal birth—one was a forceps delivery and the other the Cæsarean birth in a diabetic mother mentioned above. One microcephalic child, weighing 4 lb. 14 oz., was said by the mother to be full-time. There may have been antenatal damage. In one case there was jaundice of prematurity which led to cerebral irritation. The eventual cerebral abnormality was possibly related to the jaundice rather than to the prematurity. In one case the mother had suffered from German measles at 6 weeks and the resultant defective sight and spastic quadriplegia was possibly related to this rather than to the prematurity. In 5 cases the spastic quadriplegia was asymmetrical and there was evidence of cerebral damage. All suffered from fits later. In one case there was a known subdural hæmatoma. Four weighed over 5 lb. at birth. The overall evidence in these cases was one of cerebral catastrophe.

Finally there remain 18 interesting cases who from careful criticism appear to be examples of a symmetrical spasticity comparable to the premature group of paraplegias—a more severe involvement. The possible connexion between these two groups was noted by Asher and Schonell (1950).

They were all cases of symmetrical quadriplegia in that the condition of both legs was similar. In each case the arm of preference was better than the other. The birth weights included 3 babies under 2 lb. and 4 between 2 and 3 lb. at birth.

This group is rather ill-defined, but the overall picture is one of severe spastic quadriplegia with an intelligence within normal limits and fewer other neurological signs. Twelve children were considered educable and 3 attended a normal school. There was strabismus in 11 of the 18, a similar finding to that in the group of paraplegics.

There was no hearing loss and no sensory loss in those old enough to be tested. Two of these children were having frequent fits and 3 others gave a history of an occasional fit in infancy. Four out of 14 E.E.G.s were normal, 3 showed an interesting quiet type of record, and 7 showed instability, possibly suggesting additional cerebral damage.

Possibly in this group of 18 children prematurity is the most significant factor, although undoubtedly some had suffered specific cerebral damage—a hazard of prematurity.

Six of these children attended a special spastic school and 2 in a rural area had a home teacher. It is this type of spastic cerebral palsy for which a special unit is particularly desirable, as there is frequently evidence of good intelligence with a severe physical handicap which may improve with treatment. A number of children in this group suffered from perceptual difficulties and had peculiar difficulties in learning the three Rs, which will be discussed in a later chapter. For this reason again a special educational unit is desirable for individual help with learning difficulties.

Abnormal Delivery.—An abnormal delivery took place in no fewer than 34 cases. A difficult forceps delivery occurred 9 times, and forceps were applied in 5 further cases. There were 3 breech deliveries, in 2 of which forceps were applied.

There was one brow presentation finally delivered as a face presentation. A Cæsarean section was performed three times, in one case for fœtal distress, in one case because of the presence of Rh-antibodies, and in one case because of two previous stillbirths in a diabetic mother. There were 6 histories of multiple births, all causing prematurity.

In 6 cases there was a history of a precipitate birth at the end of a normal pregnancy. In 3 of these cases there was asphyxia with later evidence of cerebral irritation. In the other 3 cases the symptoms appeared after a few days, and in one subdural hæmatomata were diagnosed and treated.

In 3 further cases a precipitate delivery at the end of an abnormal pregnancy may have been a significant factor in the eventual cerebral pathology.

Normal Full-time Birth.—With this pronounced history of antenatal and natal disturbance in the majority of cases, it was found that only 16 cases gave a history of a normal full-time birth after a normal pregnancy. One was a case of phenyl-pyruvic oligophrenia and one child had a cleft palate and later severe physiological jaundice. Three children had severe neonatal symptoms in spite of the normal birth. In 6 cases the spastic quadriplegia was known to have followed an illness in later infancy. In 5 cases only was there no unusual history or symptom.

Neonatal Abnormalities.—*Asphyxia* occurred in 30 patients and was followed in nearly every case by symptoms of cerebral irritation in the neonatal period. In 12 cases the baby was premature and there was feeble respiratory control for some time after birth. In 5 cases the fœtal asphyxia followed a long and difficult labour, complicated in one case by pre-eclampsia. Five followed a precipitate birth in 2 of which there had been a history of A.P.H. One baby cried immediately after a normal birth and then ceased for several minutes, presumably due to poor physiological control. In 2 cases at least there was evidence of an abnormal baby responding poorly to extra-uterine life.

Jaundice occurred in 10 cases. In 3 cases there was rhesus incompatibility, antenatally diagnosed in 2 and adequately treated. The eventual brain damage must have been more serious than a basal ganglia defect as all patients were severely affected spastics. There was jaundice of prematurity in 5 cases and jaundice following asphyxia in one. Severe physiological jaundice in one full-time baby gave rise to marked cerebral irritation.

Neonatal Symptoms.—Each case of asphyxia and jaundice gave considerable evidence of neurological damage in the neonatal period in the form of either an abnormal cry, undue sleepiness, twitching, convulsions, opisthotonos, or severe difficulty with sucking. In addition to these 40 cases a further 13 gave a history of neonatal difficulties, in some cases severe. In a few of the older cases and in some of the premature babies it has been impossible to obtain a full history. Two of the tiny premature babies were born at home, and beyond the fact that they were fed with a pipette, the mother did not know of any abnormal symptoms after birth. Many more details would be desirable, particularly as these small premature symmetrical quadriplegics are of such interest.

Illness after a Few Days.—In 7 cases there was a history of normal respirations at birth and no worries for a period of a few days and then a sudden severe neonatal crisis which caused marked concern. In 3 of these cases the birth had been abnormal and in 3 it had been precipitate. In one case subdural taps were negative, but the C.S.F. obtained by lumbar puncture was blood-stained. One of these cases, *Case* 24, as described earlier, came to post-mortem. There is some evidence that all these 7 cases may be bilateral hemiplegics. The pathology may have been one of venous thrombosis, engorgement, and hæmorrhage following severe pressure on the head, leading to bilateral involvement.

No Neonatal Worries.—In marked contrast to this serious history of neonatal symptoms, there were 13 cases in which it seemed fairly certain that the baby gave no worries to the parents or attendants. In 7 of these cases the spastic quadriplegic condition dates from a later illness. In 3 of the other cases there was undoubted evidence of an abnormal baby from birth, presumably due to an antenatal cerebral maldevelopment or genetic cause. In 3 other cases the cause remains obscure. All three were educable and the condition in two was slight.

5

DISCUSSION

In this fairly large collection of 68 cases of congenital spastic quadriplegia there is an interwoven pattern of possible causes— an inherited genetic cause, an inherited cerebral instability, antenatal illness, antepartum hæmorrhage, threatened mis- carriage, pre-eclampsia, antenatal fœtal distress, a long and difficult labour, a precipitate labour, asphyxia, jaundice, pre- maturity, rhesus incompatibility. Possibly nothing but post- mortem examination can unravel all the significant factors.

ACQUIRED SPASTIC QUADRIPLEGIA

Comparable to the condition of acquired hemiplegia, 7 cases of postnatal illness fall into a distinct group of acquired spastic quadriplegia. The 7 cases therefore are described separately.

Case 26.—A second child, who after a normal birth and neonatal period was taken severely ill at one month of age with otitis media and symptoms of meningitis. He was admitted to hospital. The C.S.F. was normal and the true diagnosis was left in doubt. He developed into a case of spastic quadriplegia. At the age of 6 years he was admitted to a Spastic School and the diagnosis is now very strongly in favour of a bilateral hemiplegia. The condition of his hands is worse than his legs and there is definite astereognosis in both hands. There is defect of growth on the right side. There is defective vision of the right eye and a suggestion of a field of vision defect. His face is markedly spastic, his speech is slurred, and he cannot form his consonants with lip movement. There is evidence of slight motor aphasia, he can recognize letters and compare them, but cannot say the names. His arithmetic ability and his perception of shape seem good. In spite of these handicaps, his intelligence is normal and he will be a very interesting boy to study.

Case 27.—A third child, who after a normal birth was taken ill at 3½ months with an illness diagnosed as encephalitis. She developed into a blind, deaf, and severe spastic quadriplegic. The illness may have some relationship to the sudden catastrophe in cases of acute hemiplegia.

Case 28.—A first child, born after a postmature delivery, hastened by inductions. The evidence is not quite definite that he was normal before a serious illness at 6 months when he was circumcised. There was severe difficulty in resuscitation from the anæsthetic and the mother states the child was never the same afterwards. He developed into a severe spastic quadriplegic. The condition of his legs and left arm was severe. The sight was impaired. There was no speech and he was an imbecile.

Case 29.—A first child who was normal until 10 months of age, when he was admitted to an isolation hospital as a case of measles encephalomyelitis. Subsequently he was found to have a mild spastic condition of the legs, evidence of a stiffness and incoordination of the hands with some hyperkinesis. He understood most of the conversation around him, but at 10½ years still had no speech. He tried to make himself understood by gesture and appeared to have true motor aphasia. He attended an occupational centre and had speech therapy.

Case 30.—A third child, born after a normal birth and infancy, was admitted to hospital at 14 months with a sudden illness diagnosed as polio-encephalitis. He developed spasticity of the arms and legs and a defective speech due to spasticity of the muscles of the tongue and vocal organs. At one time his tongue was severely spastic and almost immobile. He did not speak till 9 years of age. Throughout childhood he had frequent fits. His I.Q. was 80. His improvement was remarkable and more rapid than in cases of congenital quadriplegia. By the age of 16 years he was walking about normally, his speech had a slight hesitation only, and he was starting an apprenticeship with a cabinet maker. The response to speech therapy was most gratifying.

Case 31.—The first child, born after a gestation period of 36 weeks, weighing 5 lb. 8 oz. at birth. He had difficulty in sucking at first. At 2 years of age he had a fit following a fall and had frequent fits from the age of 2 years to 5 years. At 5 years of age he was admitted to hospital with status epilepticus, and spasticity in the limbs was noted after. He did not walk again for another year. He had spasticity of both legs with wasting on the right side, and slight spasticity and astereognosis on the left side. His I.Q. was 48 and he was hyperexcitable. Possibly he was a case of epilepsy in an already damaged brain precipitating the onset of motor symptoms as suggested by Norman (1947). The slight evidence of birth difficulty may have been significant.

Case 32.—A fourth child, who suffered from meningococcal meningitis at 9 months. She had a severe spastic quadriplegia with impaired sight and hearing.

DISCUSSION

These last 7 cases are particularly interesting because in not one of them was there evidence of the typical symmetrical quadriplegia of a congenital, or in particular, a premature case. Each of these cases rather suggested a bilateral hemiplegia or an asymmetrical bilateral cerebral lesion. The movement defect in all of these children was in marked contrast to that in the premature quadriplegics, and the underlying pathology must be different. Possibly it may be true that a symmetrical quadriplegia can only occur after antenatal or natal causation, but not following a postnatal illness.

From the evidence of these 7 cases, and from other cases which followed neonatal illness in a full-time baby, there appear to be spastic quadriplegics who do not show the typical movement-pattern defect described by Little, in particular the scissors adduction of the thighs on extension. Although no two cases are alike, they suggest a diagnosis of bilateral hemiplegia. The movement defect affects the arms more than the legs, often the distal extremities more than the proximal, and often one side more than the other. Some show involuntary movements which may be associated movements. When the child attempts to use one side the other side comes into action involuntarily. Many of these cases are of low mentality and it is difficult to test sensation ; but astereognosis has been found in 2 cases, and suspected in several others. Some have shown a defect in growth on one side. Others have shown a defect in vision which is cerebral in character and may be of the nature of a visual agnosia.

Cases of spastic quadriplegia in mental deficiency hospitals which have come to post-mortem often show bilateral parieto-occipital damage, not always symmetrical. Cases of unilateral hemiplegia may show similar unilateral damage, as in *Case* 13 which had a parieto-occipital lobectomy. It seems possible that some cases of spastic quadriplegia are bilateral hemiplegics of the parieto-occipital type. In the majority of cases they are of low intelligence.

SUMMARY

A detailed description of the motor defect in spastic quadriplegia shows a wide variety of movement-pattern defects.

There is evidence in some cases of an abnormal family history of neurological conditions, suggesting a genetic factor.

Two cases were due to a congenital defect.

There is a marked history of antenatal illness and antepartum hæmorrhage associated in many cases with the birth of an ineducable child.

The statistical findings show a significant increase in the incidence of a first birth to an older mother.

The graph of birth-weights shows a bimodal pattern with a high proportion of very small birth-weights, and a higher proportion than normal of above average birth-weights.

Twenty-nine cases were premature at birth. Eighteen of these show a typical symmetrical condition of the legs. The intelligence in 12 of these cases was within normal limits ; and it is suggested that they may fit into a particular clinical syndrome comparable with the premature symmetrical paraplegics.

Thirty cases gave a history of neonatal asphyxia, and 10 of severe neonatal jaundice.

Sixty-two cases gave considerable concern in the neonatal period due to varying signs of cerebral irritation.

Seven cases followed an illness in later infancy, and their case histories are given in detail.

Only 3 gave no history of antenatal, natal, neonatal, or postnatal disturbance.

A picture is given of a severe but variable motor handicap due to a wide variety of aetiological factors.

CHAPTER IX

ATHETOSIS

WHEREAS in the other types of cerebral palsy the movement defect is one of poverty of movement, in athetosis there is a generalized excess of movement. Hammond (1881) described athetosis as "mainly characterized by an inability to retain the fingers and toes in any position in which they may be placed and by their continual motion". Kinnier Wilson (1925) variously described athetosis as "a perpetual blending of one movement into another", as "a mobile spasm, which flows indifferently into muscular units", or as "a medley of contractions entangling the limb, as it were, leading to no accomplishment".

Athetosis describes a child whose whole body passes into a state of slow, writhing, muscular contractions when attempting any voluntary movement. On attempting to use the hands, the head turns, the face grimaces, the mouth opens, both arms pass into a series of contractions, the trunk squirms, and in many cases the child cannot control the leg movements. An intelligent child may attempt to make these involuntary movements appear normal by continuously fidgeting with objects, or by destructive actions such as tearing or scribbling, to suggest that the movements are voluntary. He may be in danger of being considered a 'fidget'.

Various observers watching these children (Gesell and Amatruda, 1949; Agassiz, O'Donnell, and Collis, 1949; Bobath, B., and K., 1954) have noticed that the movement defect is associated with a derangement of the developing reflex pattern of movement. Whereas the progress in motor ability in a normal child is influenced by reflexes, such as the Moro reflex, the tonic neck reflex, the Landau reflex, the jump reflex, the body-righting reflexes, and the balance reflexes, which appear and then disappear as the child's power of movement develops, in a brain-damaged child the ordered appearance and disappearance of these normal reflexes is upset.

In particular the athetoid child may show undue persistence of the Moro or startle reflex, and the tonic neck reflex. A sudden noise will send one of these children into a severe spasm, involving the whole body, and if the child is able to stand, he may lose his balance. All athetoid children, even the mildest cases, except perhaps some who have been specially treated, will show remains of the tonic neck reflexes. (*Figs.* 24–26.) On turning the head to one side the jaw arm extends, the skull arm flexes, and in some cases the alternate leg flexes and extends due to the persistence of an asymmetrical tonic neck reflex. When the head is in mid-position, both arms are abducted and flexed at the elbows, due to the persistence of a symmetrical tonic neck reflex. These positions are shown in several photographs and can be recognized as the normal walking pattern of an athetoid. The abnormality that makes an athetoid person appear unusual, even to a layman, is that he walks with the head wobbling from one side to the other with the alternate movements of the legs. At the same time, his arms are held in the air, with elbows flexed and the flexion alternates as the child moves one leg and then the other, and has some rhythmic relationship with the movements of the head. Even the mild athetoid case attending ordinary school, whose photograph is shown in the chapter on ataxia (*Fig.* 29), shows the presence of a tonic neck reflex, and it can be observed in the other photographs of athetoid children.

The presence of this reflex, and of the Landau reflex, which holds the head in a hyperextended position, prevents an athetoid child from rolling normally from supine to prone, unless he uses his head as a lever (*Fig.* 26). The symmetric tonic neck reflexes prevent the child from being able to place his hands on the ground in a prone position and thus stop him crawling (*Fig.* 27). It has been found that some athetoid children can walk with these odd movements of the head and arms and yet be unable to roll over or crawl.

Because of the presence of tonic neck reflexes, the arms in an athetoid are often useless, and, for instance, to pick up an

object with a flexed elbow, the child must look the other way.
It is not surprising that some athetoid children have found it
easier to use their feet rather than their hands for play.   One
child at a Spastic School can play with sand with her feet,
while her arms are in such severe spasm that when she is
undressed the fingers will shoot forward in uncontrolled
spasm and scratch her chest.   It has been noted by various
observers (Agassiz and others, 1949 ; Bobath, B., and K., 1954 ;
Pohl, 1950) that these abnormal reflex patterns can be inhibited
by special training methods.   A strong tonic neck reflex on one
side can cause a scoliosis before the age of eighteen months.

In most athetoids, the normal balance reflexes are present
but cannot be brought into action.   If the child is pushed
over, he cannot put out his hands or abduct his legs to save
himself (*Fig.* 28).   The ease with which these children are
knocked over may give an impression of ataxia, particularly if
a certain amount of hypotonia is present.

The tone of the muscles in athetosis may vary from severe
spasm to apparent hypotonia, but during any movement, spasm
can always be found in some muscles and this spasm may
pass rapidly from one group of muscles to the other.   The
tone of all the body musculature is normal during sleep.

It is not always easy to distinguish between a severe tension
or hypertonic athetosis and a spastic quadriplegia, as in both
types variations may occur in the movement pattern.   In
severe extension, a tension or hypertonic athetoid may lie
with the arms in the typical athetoid position of arm abduction
and elbow flexion, but with the legs in scissors formation with
plantar flexion of the feet.   The severe tension may prevent
the athetoid movement ' getting through '.   A spastic quadriplegic will lie in a similar position in extension, often with
the arms in the same position.   The sitting position and the
position of the hands are described in the chapter on quadriplegia and may be the same in both types, and it is only the
excess of movement in the athetoid that clearly differentiates
them.   The distinction can only be made when the athetoid
is fairly relaxed and the movements ' come through '.

Again, some cases with severe spasticity in the legs may be
cases of athetosis superimposed on a spastic paraplegia.   They

PLATE XIII

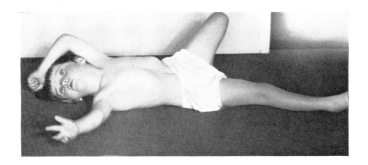

Fig. 24.

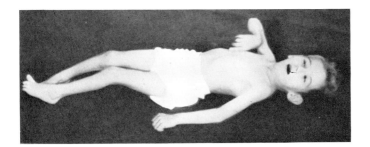

Fig. 25.

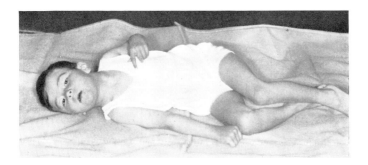

Fig. 26.

Three cases of tonic neck reflex in athetosis interfering with normal rolling.

PLATE XIV

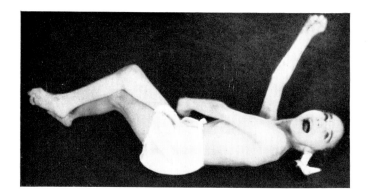

A

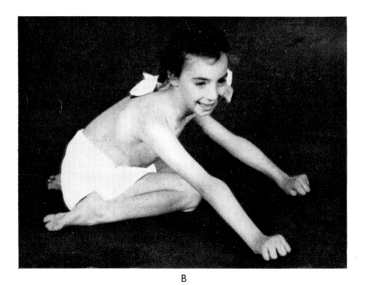

B

Fig. 27.—A case of athetosis. **A**, In extension ; **B**, In flexion.

PLATE XV

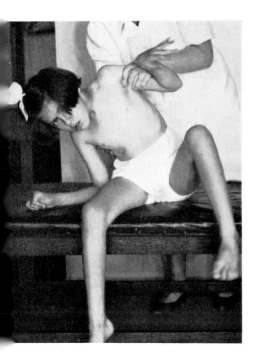
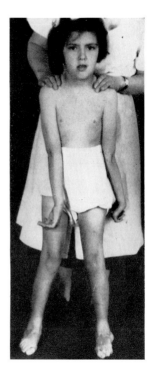

Fig. 28.—A case of athetosis showing lack of normal balance
reactions.

PLATE XVI

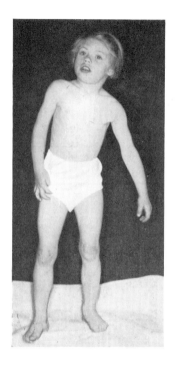
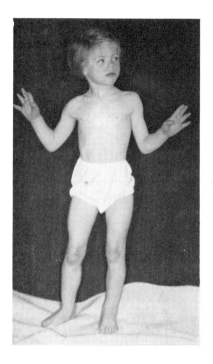

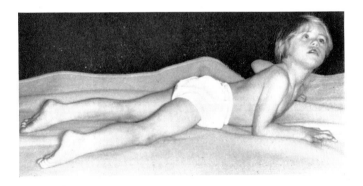

Fig. 29.—A case of athetosis attending normal school. The bizarre movements which were evidence of mild tonic neck reflexes suggested ataxia.

are included under the heading of athetosis. Four cases of hemiathetosis have been described in the chapter on hemiplegias.

Another pitfall in separating an athetoid from a severe spastic quadriplegic is the presence of associated movements in the latter, if it is in reality a case of bilateral hemiplegia. When this child attempts to move a limb there is a corresponding movement in the opposite leg or arm as in a unilateral hemiplegia. We have felt that one or two cases of spastic quadriplegia that might have been diagnosed as athetoid are of this type.

The numerical findings in the 33 cases of athetosis seen are given below :—

Family History.—
　1 father epileptic ; 1 sister monoplegic twin ; 1 abnormal second cousin.
Mother's Age at Birth.—
　Under 19, 1 ; 20–29, 15 ; 30–39, 14 ; 40+, 2 ; uncertain, 1.
Order of Pregnancy.—
　First, 16 ; second, 8 ; third, 5 ; fourth, 3 ; uncertain, 1.
Gestation Period.—
　Under 33 weeks, 10 ; 33–38 weeks, 5 ; 39–42 weeks, 16 ; over 43 weeks, 1 ; uncertain, 1.
Antenatal Abnormalities.—
　Pre-eclampsia, 7.
　A.P.H., 4.
　Membranes ruptured 1 week before, 1.
　Known Rhesus factor, 4.
　Inductions, 4.
　Rhesus factor present, not known antenatally, 3.
　Hernia, 1.
　Pyelitis, 1.
Birth Process.—
　Breech, 6.
　Forceps, 4 (1 with prolapsed cord).
　Cæsarean, 2.
　Multiple, 1.
　Precipitate labour, 4.
　Long labour, 3.
　Normal full-time birth (no Rhesus complication), 3.
Male : Female.—17 : 16.
Birth Weight.—
　Under 4 lb., 7 ; 4 lb.+, 5 ; 5 lb.+, 6 ; 6 lb.+, 8 ; 7 lb.+, 4 ; 8 lb.+, 2 ; 9 lb.+, 1.

Premature.—
    12 and 1 definite premature at 6 lb.
Neonatal Abnormalities.—
    Asphyxia, 14 ; uncertain, 3 ; jaundice, 16 ; uncertain, 3 ; cerebral
    irritation, 8 ; feeding difficulty, 10.
*Convulsions after 4 Weeks.—*8.
*Cerebral Infection in Infancy.—*1.
Visual Defect.—
    Impaired vision, 1 ; muscular imbalance, 17.
*Hearing Defect.—*12.
*Speech Defect.—*28.
*Hydrocephalus.—*1.
*Microcephalus.—*6.
Hand Dominance.—
    Only 7 were definitely right-handed.
School Placement.—
    O.S., 4 ; Spastic School, 17 ; P.H., 1 ; Deaf School, 1 ; Oc.C., 5 ;
    not yet placed, 5.

AETIOLOGY

In this distinctive type of abnormal movement defect there
does not appear to be the same wide variety of aetiological
factors. In this Bristol series there was no case suggesting
either a genetic inheritance or a congenital cerebral defect,
although such cases are reported.

Four abnormalities in the birth process or neonatal period
appeared to be the significant causal factors. Pre-eclampsia
(7 cases), prematurity (13 cases), asphyxia neonatorum (14
cases), and neonatal jaundice (16 cases) appear to be inter-
related as possible causes for the athetoid condition. One or
other of these four factors was present in 30 out of the 33
cases. In only 3 cases was there a history of a normal birth
with no significant recorded finding to account for the condition. These three births occurred at home, and birth notes
are not available.

In one case, after a breech birth with asphyxia, there was
an illness diagnosed as a possible meningitis at 6 months of
age. The significance of this last factor cannot be assessed.
In infancy, cases of athetosis show frequent spasms of head
retraction which might raise a suspicion of meningitis.

Many cases of severe athetosis have ended their lives in
institutions, and the brain has been available for post-mortem

examination. A frequent finding has been an abnormality of the corpus striatum, a condition described as *état marbré*, which is due to "the presence of myelinated fibres in aggregations of a density abnormal for that particular region of the nervous system" (Norman, 1947). The cause of this condition has been variously ascribed to a prenatal anomaly of growth (Vogt and Vogt, 1920; Alexander, 1942), or to petechial hæmorrhages from branches of the vein of Galen in cases of asphyxia (Malamud, 1950; Schwartz, 1924), or to foci of anæmic necrosis following the cutting off of oxygen (Norman, personal communication). These cases are thought to have followed neonatal asphyxia. In cases of jaundice, either due to rhesus incompatibility or other factors, the basal ganglia may also be affected, but there is more selective damage to the globus pallidus and subthalamic nuclei. But as has been shown by other observers, and is borne out in this survey, after severe neonatal jaundice there may be evidence of damage in other areas of the brain.

In some cases there is evidence of other cerebral damage. In 4 cases, after prolonged observation the children were considered to be ineducable. It has been suggested that there may be associated thalamic damage, " leading to poor development of cortical function " (Norman, personal communication). In one of these 4 cases the E.E.G. was normal, and in 2 the records were of general low amplitude, which may be significant.

There was clinical evidence of cortical damage in 3 other cases. In one child epileptiform fits had occurred, and the E.E.G. showed occasional sharp spikes. In another with severe tension athetosis and possible evidence of spasticity, the E.E.G. suggested gross abnormality. This child was of normal intelligence. In the third, the air encephalogram showed an increased subarachnoid space and width of sulci suggestive of cerebral atrophy and agenesis. This last child appeared to be a typical athetoid following an attack of white asphyxia and severe physiological jaundice with neonatal cerebral irritation.

Apart from the possible thalamic and cortical damage, a fair number of these cases show deafness. This combination of athetosis and deafness was noted first by Phelps (1941).

Perlstein (1953) states that at least 30 per cent of cases of kernicterus are deaf. This finding possibly calls for further pathological explanation. Twelve of the present series were deaf, or partially deaf, and 3 were ineducable ; the deafness may have been part of the gross brain pathology. However, 5 cases fell very clearly into the syndrome described by Perlstein and Phelps. The children showed athetosis, defective upward movement of the eyes, and deafness. The athetosis was somewhat different in pattern from other cases in that there was little tension and poor head control and consequently the children appeared almost ataxic. The deafness took the form of a high-frequency deafness, although in 4 cases it was severe. The intelligence in all these children was good and the children were described as ' triers '. The 4 E.E.G.s taken were normal. This syndrome of athetosis, high-frequency deafness, and defective upward movement of the eyes is considered to be due to a lesion involving the superior colliculus and cochlear nucleus.

The combination of athetosis and deafness appears to follow neonatal jaundice more frequently than neonatal asphyxia. Some cases have been due to rhesus incompatibility. Others have followed severe physiological jaundice with kernicteric symptoms. They were not cases of ABO incompatibility, and the exact aetiology has not yet been unravelled.

Seven of the cases have followed jaundice of extreme prematurity. All weighed 4 lb. or under at birth. The possible relationship of this condition to vitamin K administration has been discussed by Laurance (1955) and Meyer and Angus (1956). Doses of the order of 10 mg., t.d.s. for 5 days had been administered to at least 5 of the cases. With new techniques of repeated exchange transfusions for raised serum bilirubin in the neonatal period, cases of athetosis due to these three causes may cease to occur.

Deafness may be associated with severe, mild, or no athetosis, and alternatively, marked athetosis may occur with severe, slight, or no deafness. For the last few months cases of athetosis are presenting for special education of a slightly different pattern from the more hypertonic post-asphyxial athetoids of older age-groups. They give this history of jaundice of prematurity, or jaundice due to rhesus incompatibility, and throughout their school life they will be a special educational problem with the double handicap of athetosis and deafness.

Visual, auditory, speech, and sensory defects and fits are discussed in separate chapters.

Air encephalograms have been obtained in 3 cases—one was abnormal, as already mentioned, and 2 were normal.

DISCUSSION

This group of athetoid children is somewhat more sharply separated from the other types of brain-injured children by the type of movement handicap and by the cerebral pathology. The aetiology varies, although in every case there is clinical evidence of basal ganglia damage. This group, on the whole, is more homogeneous than the other groups of movement defects.

SUMMARY

Thirty-three cases of athetosis are discussed.

The movement defect with the fluctuating tone in the muscles, the abnormal movements, and the upset of normal reflex movement pattern is similar in every case.

Nearly all cases appear to date from an abnormality in the birth process or neonatal period, and there is little conclusive evidence that a case has developed following a post-neonatal illness, or has had a genetic causation.

The cerebral damage is presumably in the region of the basal ganglia.

A few cases show, in addition, evidence of cortical damage, and there is a possibility of thalamic damage.

Five cases showed a definite syndrome of ataxic athetosis, defective upward movement of the eyes, and high-frequency deafness.

The combination of athetosis and deafness following prematurity and neonatal jaundice is discussed.

CHAPTER X

ATAXIA

IN all accounts of cerebral palsy, space is given to this group and the incidence is suggested as being 1 per cent (Asher and Schonell, 1950), 3 per cent (Evans, 1948 b), 7·23 per cent (Ingram and Kerr, 1954), and 8 per cent (Pohl, 1950). On carefully analysing the 301 cases that have attended the Bristol Cerebral Palsy Assessment Clinic, it has been found increasingly difficult to decide what is meant by ataxia. It seems fairly certain that cases of true cerebellar ataxia in childhood are rarely seen. A case of hereditary cerebellar ataxia with spasticity as described by Ford (1944) was not found, and he states that he has never seen a case of cerebellar ataxia due to birth injury. The cerebellar syndrome as described by Monrad Krohn (1948) of hypotonia, asthenia, decomposition of movements, dysmetria, rebound phenomena, dysdiadochokinesia, and past pointing was not encountered. On the other hand, as pointed out by Norman (personal communication), children with cerebellar defects do not show the same symptoms as adults, and cases have come to post-mortem with severe congenital atrophy of the cerebella, which in life presented as cases of spastic quadriplegia with idiocy. Norman also states that he has not met a case of damaged cerebellum as the sole defect at post mortem in a cerebral palsied child. This finding is surprising and may cut across preconceived ideas of neonatal anoxic damage to the brain, as it is known that the Purkinje cells of the cerebellum are particularly sensitive to anoxia.

It seems plain that in the cases of ataxia described here and elsewhere we are not dealing with true cerebellar ataxia. In fact, Perlstein (1953) says that ataxia can occur after a lesion in the frontal cortex. Some cases described as ataxia in the past may have been very mild cases of spasticity or athetosis.

A mild spastic child, in a state of slight flexor spasm, with knees and hips flexed, head poked forward, and shoulders retracted, may have a shuffling gait and be easily knocked over, and with the absence of ability to balance may appear like an ataxic child. A mild athetoid child who walks with the head turned to one side, arms raised and flexed at the elbows, with incoordination of the legs, may appear to be ataxic, using the arms for balance. It can be shown on careful examination, however, that this odd position of the head and arms is the remains of a tonic neck reflex, and does not serve a useful purpose, such as assisting balance (*Fig.* 29).

There is a possibility that some cases described as ataxias would more correctly fall under the definition of apraxia as described by Russell Brain (1955) and Macdonald Critchley (1953 b). Apraxia is an inability to carry out willed movements. Critchley describes various disorders of motility due to damaged parietal lobes. The abnormal movement pattern in some of these ataxic children may have an origin in parietal lobe pathology, particularly as some of them showed perceptual and learning difficulties suggestive of parietal lobe damage.

Phelps (1941) describes ataxia as an inability to direct normally initiated motion. This inability is not associated with spasticity or flaccidity. In this chapter it is proposed to discuss all the odd types of cerebral palsy which do not demonstrate spasticity or athetosis, but which have a definite cerebral palsy of an incoordinated type. Some cases do show hypotonia.

There were 29 cases. The numerical findings are given below, but as this is so obviously a mixed clinical group they have only slight significance.

Family History of Neurological Abnormality.—8 cases.
Age of Mother.—
    Under 20, 1 ; 20–29, 15 ; 30–39, 11 ; 40+, 1 ; uncertain, 1.
Order of Birth.—
    First, 17 ; second, 7 ; third, 3 ; fourth, 2.
Gestation Period.—
    Under 33, 1 ; 33–38, 6 ; 39–42, 18 ; over 43, 3 ; uncertain, 1.
Birth Process.—
    Antenatal abnormality :
        A.P.H., 1 ; hydramnios, 1 ; syphilis, treated, 1 ; severe shock, 1 ;
        antipertussis injection at 5/12, 1 ; antibodies present, 1 ;

pre-eclampsia, 6 ; induction of labour, 7 ; forceps, 5 ; precipitate, 1 ; long labour, 2 ; normal full-time birth, 14.

Male : Female.—18 : 11.

Birth Weights.—

Under 4 lb., 2 ; 4 lb.+, 2 ; 5 lb.+, 4 ; 6 lb.+, 8 ; 7 lb.+, 7 ; 8 lb.+, 2 ; 9 lb.+, 4.

Premature.—6.

Neonatal Abnormalities.—

Asphyxia, 7 ; jaundice, 3 ; signs of cerebral irritation, 3 ; feeding difficulties, 8.

Convulsions after 4 Weeks.—9.

Cerebral Infection or Catastrophe.—2.

Visual Defects.—

Impaired vision, 7 ; muscular imbalance, 12.

Hearing Defects.—0.

Speech Defects.—5.

Hydrocephalus.—9.

Microcephalus.—5.

School Placement.—

O.S., 8 ; Spastic School, 5 ; P.H., 4 ; E.S.N., 6 ; Oc.C., 2 ; not yet placed, 4.

In discussing these 29 cases under their clinical patterns, they appear to fall roughly into the following groups.

GROUP 1. HEREDITARY ATAXIA

In this group there were 7 cases which are discussed very briefly.

Case 33.—A case of Friedreich's ataxia with the additional lesion, frequently seen, of heart disease. She is included in the survey only because she was presented as a case of cerebral palsy. Post-mortem findings showed brain-stem damage, particularly of the globus pallidus, subthalamic nuclei, and dentate nuclei.

Case 34.—Had two older brothers, both of whom had died in a mental deficiency colony. One of these boys had been severely jaundiced at birth. There was no evidence of rhesus incompatibility in the mother at the patient's birth, but the labour was induced 4 weeks early to prevent kernicterus. He was born after a normal birth, weighing 6 lb. 8 oz., and gave no trouble in the neonatal period. He was a hypotonic, incoordinated child with marked pes planus. He did not walk until 30 months of age and then only after prolonged physiotherapy. His hypotonia persisted. The spine radiograph showed spina bifida occulta only. His I.Q. was 75 and he later attended a school for educationally subnormal pupils.

Case 35.—Born after a normal birth, weighing 7 lb. 5 oz. There were no neonatal worries. He walked at 12 months, but always unsteadily and on a wide base. His arms and legs were held rigidly at times, and a tremor had been noted at 4 years of age. The plantar reflexes were flexor. The E.E.G. was abnormal showing " sharp and slow discharges from the posterior region ". He later attended ordinary school and had an I.Q. of 106, but his odd ataxic walk was still present at 6 years. The only suggestive history was that his father had been rejected from the army because of ' claw toes '.

Case 36.—Born after a normal birth, weighing 6 lb. 8 oz. The family had been ' bombed out ' 10 days before his birth. He was referred at the age of 11 years because of clumsy movements, particularly in writing. He was a thin asthenic type, left-eyed and right-handed. There was a marked tremor in his hands, which interfered with all his movements. An occasional stammer was present. The plantar responses were flexor, but there was marked pes cavus in both feet, with severe dorsiflexion of the big toes. The jerks were normal and the abdominal reflexes present. The radiograph of the skull and the E.E.G. were normal. His I.Q. was 80. He was the brother of *Case* 37.

Case 37.—A hypotonic ataxic child, born after normal delivery and weighing 6 lb. 12 oz. He had pes planus and eversion of the feet and did not walk until 3½ years old. Toilet training and speech were normal. His I.Q. was 100, and the E.E.G., C.S.F., A.E.G., and radiograph of the skull were normal.

Finally, included in this group are the following 2 cases, which are particularly interesting types of incoordination and fall outside the normal pattern of motor handicap, in that the true defect was sensory in nature.

Case 38.—An only child, born after a normal delivery, weighing 7 lb. Her movement handicap necessitated her attendance at a physically handicapped school from the age of 5 years to 11 years. She walked alone but badly at 20 months, but was unable to feed herself until 5 years of age. Owing to her own perseverance she was eventually transferred to a Grammar School, and after taking the General Certificate of Education took a nursery nurse's course. She was first seen by the Assessment Team at the age of 17 years. Her movement handicap was then very slight, and was not apparently noticeable to close friends. On examination there was an awkwardness in her hand movements. She tended to hyperextend the fingers and pronate the wrists. The shoulder and elbow movements were slightly stiff only. Her left hand was worse than her right. The knee-jerks were slightly exaggerated. There was no clonus and the plantar reflexes were flexor. After examination it was found that the defect was sensory in nature. There was astereognosis and loss of sense of position in both hands. The girl had realized this herself and used her visual powers to control her hands when typing or playing the piano. Considering her early history, with delay in reaching the milestones of motor development, she had mastered this method of control very successfully. The family history in this case was interesting. She stated that she had two paternal cousins, not siblings, with the same handicap.

This interesting case naturally stimulated a search for a further case, and one other was found, *Case* 39, which had previously been noted as not fitting into any normal movement-pattern defect.

Case 39.—The first-born of an apparent full-time twin pregnancy, weighing 4 lb. 13 oz. at birth. There was slight neonatal jaundice, and feeding difficulties. He did not walk until 2 years of age. His speech was normal. There was a bilateral internal strabismus dating from 10 months of age. He was left-handed and left-eyed. His only movement upset, at 5 years, was an unusual motor incoordination of the hands, which were almost choreic in nature with hyperextension of the fingers and pronation of the wrists. His legs appeared normal and the plantar responses flexor. A later examination revealed an astereognosis and loss of sense of position in the hands. The sense of vibration and touch were normal. His I.Q. was 87+ and there were no perceptual difficulties. The electroencephalogram suggested an involvement of the cortex anterior to the right occipital lobe and towards the right temporal area.

With the absence of a family history, it seems difficult to decide whether this is a case of hereditary defect as *Case* 38 above, or whether in view of the birth history and the E.E.G. the condition was due to brain trauma in the region of the parietal lobes.

GROUP 2.   ATAXIA FOLLOWING ABNORMAL BIRTHS

In the second group there were 8 cases that appeared to follow birth trauma, and short case histories are given on the opposite page.

These 8 cases briefly tabulated represent a group of inco-ordinated children with intelligence below normal. In each case there is suggestive evidence of birth trauma, although as in most cases, the evidence of cerebral damage at birth can only be circumstantial. It may be, however, that there are other cases of awkward backward children in school with a suggestive history of birth trauma. This rather indeterminate group of 'cerebral palsy' cases cannot, therefore, be considered complete.

CASE No.	BIRTH WEIGHT	BIRTH PROCESS	NEONATAL SYMPTOMS	MOVEMENT UPSET	I.Q.
40	8 lb.	Pre-eclampsia; gestation 43 weeks; duration of labour 90 hours; forceps	None mentioned	Walked at nearly 3 years of age; talked at 4½ years; generally incoordinated; plantars flexor	Ineducable
41	5 lb. 12 oz.	B.B.A. blue asphyxia	Feeding difficulties	General incoordination in both hands noticed for 3 years; hypotonic, easily knocked over; E.E.G. within normal range; left plantar, extensor response	86
42	6 lb. 1 oz.	Gestation 36 weeks; normal birth	Collapsed at 48 hours; in oxygen tent 4 days; feeding difficulties	Left internal strabismus; dribbling until 6 years; generally incoordinated gait	80+
43	3 lb.	Precipitate delivery at 34 weeks' gestation	White asphyxia; jaundice	Hands clumsy, difficulty at 7½ years with stair climbing	79
44	7 lb.	Medical induction; normal delivery	Hæmatemesis at 2 days—transfusion	Marked incoordination of hands; right ankle clonus; toneless staccato speech; strabismus and impaired vision; A.E.G. shows porencephaly; stiff jerky gait—easily knocked over	95
45	4 lb. 9½ oz.	Medical induction for severe pre-eclampsia; normal birth	Sucked badly	Incoordinated microcephalic; walked at 30 months, pes planus; one convulsion in infancy	65
46	5 lb.	Mother treated for syphilis during pregnancy; gestation 36 weeks	Blue asphyxia; oxygen tent and intravenous feeds	Stiff incoordinated walk; plantar flexor; walked at 30 months	Below normal
47	5 lb. 7 oz.	Severe pre-eclampsia; normal birth	White asphyxia; in oxygen tent	Generally incoordinated; walked at 22 months; abnormal E.E.G.	62

GROUP 3. ATAXIA FOLLOWING JAUNDICE

Severe neonatal jaundice, whether due to rhesus incompatibility or other factors, is a frequent cause of cerebral irritation with opisthotonos and twitching in the neonatal period. In some cases the cerebral damage is permanent and these cases have been grouped under the heading of kernicterus. The pathology shows pigmentation of and necrosis in brain-cells. The pigmentation and cerebral damage may be widespread, but are usually most marked in the basal ganglia. For this reason the most frequent movement upset in a cerebrally damaged child after neonatal jaundice is athetosis, but it is not surprising, as with all these cases of cerebral palsy, that other movement upsets are seen as well.

Two cases of ataxia following neonatal jaundice have been encountered.

Case 48.—The second child, born after a full-time normal delivery, weighing 5 lb. 12 oz. at birth. There was severe neonatal jaundice with cerebral irritation for 10 days. She has a bilateral internal strabismus dating from birth, treated by operation. She walks like a blind child and has difficulty in focusing. Her movement upset is illustrated in *Fig.* 31. She walks with head, hips, and knees flexed on a wide base with pes planus. The E.E.G. is abnormal and is suggestive of an abnormality of the posterior regions of both hemispheres, also involving deep structures. There are occasional spikes from the right temporal area.

Case 49.—Born postmaturely, after maternal pre-eclampsia, weighing 9 lb. 2 oz. at birth. The pregnancy was complicated by the known presence of maternal antibodies due to the rhesus factor. There was slight neonatal jaundice only and he received no special treatment, but the child gave other neonatal worries, and suffered from atelectasis and feeding difficulties. At 2 years he had only just begun to walk, his muscles were flaccid, and his walk incoordinated. Speech was delayed. At 3½ years his walk was still jerky and incoordinated. There was no evidence of spasticity or athetosis, and no evidence of upset in the movement reflexes. He still had no speech and dribbled profusely, and may be a case of congenital suprabulbar palsy as described by Worster-Drout (1953). He understood what was said to him, and could feed himself with a spoon and fork. There was an internal strabismus dating from birth. He appeared to be a case of ataxia, and whether the hæmolytic diseases of rhesus origin had caused brain pathology is conjectural.

GROUP 4. ATAXIA INVOLVING HYDROCEPHALUS

A further interesting group of incoordinated children was made up of 9 hydrocephalics of differing types. They all showed hypotonia with incoordination of the legs (*Fig.* 31). There was a tendency to walk on a wide base with flat feet. Sometimes the hypotonicity was reinforced by a rigidity and a sensation of plasticity was obtained. No true spasticity (except perhaps in one case) with a stretch reflex was present. There was general incoordination of the hands and in 4 cases

Case No.	Birth Weight	Birth Details and Illnesses	Milestones and Present Condition	Investigations	I.Q.
50	2 lb. 8 oz.	Gestation 32 weeks Two attacks of meningism with xanthochromia in C.S.F. at 2 years	Walked alone with pes planus and ataxia at 5 years	—	100
51	6 lb. 8 oz.	Long labour ; forceps White asphyxia ; normal child ; hydrocephalus developed at 4 years of age	Age 9½ years C.C.* 25 in. ; impaired vision ; nystagmus ; hands incoordinated ; walks with support only ; hips internally rotated, knees flexed, pes planus	W.R. and Kahn — Toxoplasmosis — E.E.G. abnormal	62
52	7 lb. 12 oz.	Low forceps Bulging fontanelle and vomiting in neonatal period	Coarse nystagmus to right ; left internal strabismus ; slow speech ; walks with support ; flaccid on wide base, right leg slightly wasted At 2 years 10 months C.C. 19¼ in.	Radiograph of skull N.A.D. E.E.G. wave and spike A.E.G. communicating hydrocephalus	74
53	8 lb. 1 oz.	Medical induction; forceps Feeding difficulty	2 years 6 months C.C. 20 in. ; occasional nystagmus ; papilloedema at 3 years ; very flaccid ataxic walk ; coarse tremor upper limbs	Lange curve — Radiograph, large vault Ventriculography showed subarachnoid space unusually capacious ; ventricles equal in size ; defective absorption of C.S.F.	112
54	10 lb. 8 oz.	Meningitis at 3 months Hydrocephalus noted and increased until 10 months	5 years 6 months C.C. 24¾ in. ; incoordinated hands ; plasticity of legs ; unable to walk ; evidence of precocious puberty	—	83+ No learning difficulties
55	6 lb.	Hydrocephalus noted from 5 months	Impaired sight ; nystagmus ; tremor in hands ; legs plastic ; incoordinated, cannot walk alone	Died at 10 years P.M., absent septum pellucidum	80+
56	6 lb.	Premature persistent occipito posterior, forceps Feeding difficulty	Hydrocephalus as a baby ; A.F. closed at 3 years ; general incoordination	E.E.G. abnormal	93 Severe learning difficulties did mirror writing
57	7 lb.	Normal birth Hydrocephalus developed at 6 months, treated by operation	3 years 1 month C.C. 21½ in. Strabismus ; tremor in hands ; ataxia ; some general spasticity of legs ; fits	E.E.G. sharp and slow waves	97
58	10 lb.	Slight feeding difficulty	1 year 10 months C.C. 19⅞ in. General incoordination with marked hypotonicity and pes planus ; ataxic gait still noticeable at 5 years	Radiograph of skull, N.A.D. Spine, slight dorsal scoliosis to left E.E.G. aggressive in type	83

* Cranial circumference.

there was a tremor on effort.   Two of these, *Cases* 52 and 53, could have passed as cases of true cerebellar ataxia if investigation, including an air encephalogram, had not revealed an internal hydrocephalus.   In *Case* 53 particularly, the hypotonia was extreme, but a communicating hydrocephalus with widening of the subarachnoid space and defective absorption of cerebrospinal fluid was shown at operation.   This condition was presumed to be due to birth injury.   The finding of a congenital condition of internal hydrocephalus with symmetrical dilatation of the third and lateral ventricles was a surprise in the little girl (*Case* 52) and it may be that other cases of ataxia might reveal this condition.

GROUP 5.   ATAXIA FROM UNKNOWN CAUSE

To conclude the survey of this heterogeneous collection of ataxic children, short histories are given of 3 cases where the cause was unknown.

Case 59.—Born normally, with a birth weight of 6 lb. 8 oz.   She had severe infantile eczema and was in hospital for the first year of life.   At the age of 1 year she had an illness with unconsciousness for 4 days.   The C.S.F. was normal and a diagnosis was not made.   At 3 years she presented as a case of ataxia with flaccidity and incoordination.   She had not walked at 5 years, and although she appeared to understand what was said to her, she had no speech.   There may have been a motor aphasia or a general incoordination of the muscles involved in speech.   Her I.Q. was 78.

Case 60.—Born after a normal birth, weighing 7 lb. 10 oz.   A bilateral internal strabismus was present from birth.   She had difficulties with chewing and swallowing and had a monotonous, incoordinated speech.   She did not walk until 10 years of age and then walked unsteadily with a wide base and with difficulty in keeping to a line.   There was slight tremor of her hands controlled by a rigidity.   The abdominal reflexes were absent and the right plantar response extensor.   She resembled a case of Parkinsonism, with an expressionless face.   An E.E.G. showed a tendency to petit mal attacks.   Presumably she had a pathological condition of the basal ganglia.

Case 61.—Born after a normal birth, birth weight 7 lb. 12 oz.   His brother was mentally backward.   The child showed general incoordination, with odd rigid spasms of the hands.   His I.Q. was 50.

SUMMARY

Twenty-nine cases of ataxia are described.

The motor defect is one of general incoordination often with hypotonia.

The condition seen in children is not a true cerebellar ataxia, but may be caused by widespread cerebral pathology.

Seven cases appeared to be genetically determined.

Eight cases appeared to follow birth trauma.

Two cases followed neonatal jaundice.

Nine cases of ataxia were associated with hydrocephalus.

In 3 cases no aetiological cause for the condition could be found.

CHAPTER XI

RIGIDITY

WITH the present widespread interest in cerebral palsy, cases are being included in cerebral palsy surveys that in the past would have been considered as mental defectives. Many of these cases show a disorder of movement which can only be described as rigidity ; and some of these cases give a history of abnormality in the antenatal or intranatal period. In many cases the original cause of the movement upset appears to be a brain damage, and it is justifiable to include such cases under the heading of cerebral palsy.

Kinnier Wilson (1925) describes decerebrate rigidity as a condition of rigidity which is present both with passive lengthening and shortening of the limb, and with the maintenance of different postures. He suggests that lesions in different parts of the nervous system have at one or other time apparently been responsible for similar types of pathological movement. Phelps (1949) describes it as a sustained non-voluntary contractibility and loss of elasticity, an exaggeration of plastic tone, and states that rigidity may be transitory. Collis (1954) describes a condition of " variable rigidity ", in which this sense of rigidity is present at some examinations and not at others.

These cases of rigidity have not, therefore, a true stretch reflex in the muscles, but the rigidity is present throughout the manipulation of the limb, whether it is moved slowly or fast, and whether the muscles are shortened or lengthened. The extent of the rigidity appears to vary. In some children it may have been very noticeable in infancy, and may become less apparent when the child eventually learns to walk. In some cases the rigidity appears more marked around the shoulder and pelvic girdles, and these children later walk on a wide base, with a shuffling gait that in the past has been thought typical of mentally defective children.

The abnormality of movement and muscle tone in this type of cerebral palsy was studied by Norman (1933) at Stoke Park Colony. He noted that these cases showed increased tendon reflexes in 31 per cent of cases, frequently with patellar and ankle clonus. There was diminished voluntary power, a varying degree of rigidity, and an awkwardness in relaxation, with an inability to ' go loose ' rather than a true spasticity. There was often a tendency to adopt an attitude of general flexion. He considered that many of these cases were due to a developmental defect of the phylogenetically more recent part of the nervous system—the supragranular layer. He suggested that the abnormal posture and movement of a ' rigid ' mental defective was produced by the action of lower motor centres released from higher cortical control by the impairment of the supragranular cortex.

The rigidity in these cases is thus of varying severity and the most severe cases show true decerebrate rigidity.* A factor which was present in all the rigidity cases described is mental deficiency, not one case was found to be educable. But again, as suggested by Kinnier Wilson, we may be dealing with a wide selection of clinical entities.

The clinical findings are given below in the 28 cases seen.

Family History of Mental Deficiency in Close Relative.—5.
Mother's Age.—
    Under 20, 0 ; 20–29, 11 ; 30–40, 13 ; 40+, 1 ; uncertain, 3.
Order of Pregnancy.—
    First, 14 ; second, 8 ; third, 3 ; fourth+, 2 ; uncertain, 1.
Gestation Period.—
    Under 33, 0 ; 33–38 weeks, 8 ; 39–42 weeks, 20 ; uncertain, 0.
Birth Process.—
    Pre-eclampsia, 6.
    Antenatal abnormality :
        Threatened miscarriage, 4.   .
        Exophthalmic goitre, 1
        Illness, 1.
        Shock, 1.
        German measles, 1.
        Hydramnios, 2.

---

* Severe cases lie in bed rigidly flexed in a fœtal position, in contrast to cases of spastic quadriplegia who, when awake, lie in bed fully extended, often with scissors formation of the legs.

Breech delivery, 2.
Forceps, 3.
Cæsarean, 1.
Multiple, 2.
Long labour, 5.
Normal full-time birth, 19 (of these 9 showed neonatal difficulties).
Male : Female.—15 : 13.
Congenital Defects.—10.
　Spinal nævus, 2.
　Abnormal skull and sternum, 3.
　Micrognathus, 1.
　Congenital dislocation of hip, 1.
　Abnormal tiny feet, 1.
　Hypospadias, 1.
　Accessory auricle, 1.
Birth Weights.—
　Under 4 lb., 1 ; 4 lb.+, 3 ; 5 lb.+, 3 ; 6 lb.+, 6 ; 7 lb.+, 8 ;
　　8 lb.+, 5 ; 9 lb.+, 1 ; uncertain, 1.
Premature.—6.
Neonatal Abnormalities.—
　Asphyxia, 7.
　Jaundice, 3.
　Cerebral irritation, 8.
Convulsions after 4 Weeks.—17.
Cerebral Infection.—1.
Visual Defects.—
　Blind, 5.
　Impaired, 5.
　Muscular imbalance, 10.
Hearing Defect.—Impossible to test.
Speech Defect.—28, all due to mental deficiency.
Hydrocephalus.—0.
Microcephalus.—15.

AETIOLOGICAL FACTORS

HEREDITARY OR DEVELOPMENTAL CAUSE

In 2 cases the conditions which presented as rigidities were examples of known genetic diseases. One was a case of amaurotic family idiocy, Tay Sachs disease in a Jewish child, with a typical cherry-red spot at the macula. The other was a case of phenylpyruvic oligophrenia, aged 6 years, and thus considered too old to benefit by dietetic treatment.

In 5 cases there was a history of mental deficiency in a near relative. In one severe case 7 children had died in a family of 12, and one at least was known to the team, and was similar to the patient. He was a mentally defective rigid child, who had no sense of pain and had bitten away his lower lip, and unless prevented, chewed his hands. The cerebral pathology must be grossly abnormal.

The high incidence of associated congenital defects emphasized the possible genetic or developmental causation.

ANTENTAL DISTURBANCE

An interesting finding was the high proportion of cases with a history of antenatal disturbance, 10 in all. In one case there was a known history of German measles in the 7th month of pregnancy. In 2 cases the child was one of twins, the other twin weighing considerably more at birth, and being normal. As there appeared to be no evidence of birth damage, and the children gave an impression of abnormality from birth, one presumes that there may have been some defect in vascular supply to the abnormal twin. Microcephaly was present in 9 cases.

In another case the mother who had rheumatic heart disease had had two previous abnormal premature children, presumably due to placental insufficiency throughout pregnancy.

ABNORMALITY OF BIRTH PROCESS

In only 2 cases did one feel justified in assuming that cerebral trauma had occurred at birth.

Case 62.—Born at 34 weeks' gestation period after a pregnancy complicated by threatened miscarriage at the 3rd and 4th months. There was a long labour, and the child was delivered by forceps because the fœtal heart could not be heard. There was white asphyxia and signs of cerebral irritation at a few days of age. Convulsions occurred at age 7 months for one month. The C.S.F. at birth showed increased globulin. In infancy she gave the impression of blind spastic idiocy, but as she got older there was marked improvement. Her power to focus improved, until it was obvious she could see quite well, in spite of the appearances of optic atrophy. There was hypertonia of a quadriplegic pattern, but the movement upset appeared to be more of a rigid nature. She had a gross scoliosis which was due to spasm only and could be corrected. There was subluxation of her left hip due to the hypertonia. She was very late in talking but understood what was said to her to a limited degree. She was exceptionally musical and could sing or pick out on the piano about 100 tunes at 5 years of age. The E.E.G. showed abnormality in the right temporo-occipital areas, and in later years slow delta waves from the frontal areas.

Case 63.—Born after a normal pregnancy at 38 weeks, weighing 5 lb. 4 oz. The neonatal period gave the attending midwife much concern. The infant later appeared generally rigid, almost Parkinsonian in type. There was an intention tremor of the hands. The knee-jerks were exaggerated. There was no clonus and the plantar reflexes were flexor. He did not walk until 32 months of age. His face was expressionless and his speech defective. After a period at ordinary school and then at E.S.N. school, he was found to be ineducable. The E.E.G. showed continuous activity in the theta bands, indicative of deep-seated organic disturbance.

NEONATAL DISTURBANCE

Another interesting finding is the number of cases showing mild or severe symptoms of cerebral upset in the neonatal period after a normal full-time birth. There were 7 such cases. One was in the child with phenylpyruvic oligophrenia, and one in the case born after German measles in the 7th month of pregnancy. The other 5 cases all had congenital defects—one a dislocated hip, one a spinal nævus with abnormal growth of hair, one hypertelorism with an abnormality of the sternum, one a microcephaly with closed fontanelle at birth, and one with hypospadias. These findings rather suggest that an abnormal child may respond badly to the difficult process of birth and that he is poorly fitted for the sudden adjustment to extra-uterine life.

ILLNESS IN LATER INFANCY

Lastly, 2 cases occurred after an illness in later infancy.

Case 64.—The second child, born after a normal delivery, weighing 9 lb. 6 oz. at birth. There was evidence that she was a normal child until 1 year of age. She then had a severe illness, with convulsions, diagnosed as encephalitis, which appeared to be associated in time with diphtheria immunizations. From that time, she became a blind rigid idiot.

Case 65.—The first child, born after a period of pre-eclampsia, medical and surgical inductions, and a long labour, by forceps delivery. There were severe neonatal difficulties. He developed normally in every way until 5 years of age. He then had an illness diagnosed as influenza, and a movement upset was noted afterwards. The left arm, left leg, right leg, and right arm were progressively involved, and a condition of rigidity developed. There was a strabismus, and a marked scoliosis, and some urinary incontinence. There was a progressive sensory loss of temperature sensation, sense of position, and astereognosis. His intelligence was deteriorating. The E.E.G., C.S.F., and A.E.G. were normal. The exact pathology of this condition is uncertain, but Courville (1950) suggests in cases of this type that there may be a causal relationship between the neonatal anoxia and the later cerebral degeneration. He states that " necrobiotic changes (at birth) may result in functional and later structural changes only after a period of months or years ".

SUMMARY

The distinctive motor defect in rigidity is described.

Some of these cases may be due to a developmental defect in the supragranular layer of the cerebral cortex and are comparable to the type of rigid, often epileptic, mental defective seen in mental deficiency hospitals.

There was a high incidence of associated congenital defects, and in 5 cases a family history of mental deficiency.

In 10 cases there was a history of antenatal illness.

Two cases were examples of known genetic conditions.

In 2 cases birth trauma appeared to be the aetiological factor.

Two cases followed a cerebral catastrophe in later childhood.

All were ineducable.

CHAPTER XII

NUMERICAL SIGNIFICANCE OF ABNORMALITIES IN THE BIRTH PROCESS

FOLLOWING on the figures in the previous chapters an attempt was made to show the exact significance of the various birth factors in the cases where the cerebral palsy appeared to be associated with birth trauma (*Table III*). In other words, all definite hereditary cases, and cases due to a known congenital defect, and all acquired (postnatal) cases were omitted, and the numerical findings calculated on these reduced figures.

Table III.—PERCENTAGE INCIDENCE OF BIRTH ABNORMALITIES IN SIGNIFICANT CASES

TYPE	NO. OF CASES	FIRST BORN	ANTENATAL ILLNESS	HÆMORRHAGE DURING PREGNANCY	PRE-ECLAMPSIA	FORCEPS	BREECH	NORMAL BIRTH FULL-TIME	PREMATURE	ASPHYXIA	JAUNDICE	OTHER NEONATAL SYMPTOMS
		Per cent	Per cent	Per cent	Per cent	Per cent	Per cent	Per cent	Per cent	Per cent	Per cent	Per cent
Paraplegia	19	42	11	47	21	5	5	5	74	32	26	53
Monoplegia	13	38	0	0	7	7	0	46	46	7	7	14
Hemiplegia	65	52	6	15	20	25	12	24	20	32	6	46
Quadriplegia	67	46	13	15	10	20	4	16	42	43	15	64
Athetosis	33	48	10	12	21	21	18	9	39	42	48	55
Ataxia	25	64	12	7	20	12	0	48	24	24	8	48
Rigidity	24	42	8	21	17	8	8	58	25	25	13	58

As has been shown, these figures may underestimate the significance of birth abnormalities in the eventual development of cerebral palsy as some acquired cases gave a history of an abnormal birth which was possibly significant.

The numbers in these cases are small and cannot be considered statistically worth analysis. They show a high incidence of antenatal illness in the quadriplegias and rigidities, and of uterine hæmorrhage during pregnancy in the paraplegias and hemiplegias. The incidence of pre-eclampsia is high in the hemiplegias and somewhat high in athetoids and ataxias.

The incidence of breech deliveries is high in hemiplegias and athetoids.

Less than 50 per cent of the cases were born after a normal full-time birth following a normal pregnancy in every movement-defect group except the rigidities.

There is a high incidence of prematurity in all groups, but this is lowest in the rigidities.

The incidence of neonatal asphyxia is particularly high in the athetoids and quadriplegias, whereas the figure for neonatal jaundice is considerably above the other groups in the case of athetoids.

All groups show strong evidence of neonatal illness. This is least marked in the monoplegic cases.

The overall evidence is that where the cerebral palsy is not due to a known clinical or hereditary disease, the significance of an abnormal birth history is very marked.

SOCIAL GROUPS

Another interesting set of figures is produced from a study of social grouping. The following table shows the comparative incidence in the Registrar-General's Social Groups I–V of cerebral palsy cases and in controls. (*Table IV.*)

Table IV.—PERCENTAGE INCIDENCE OF CEREBRAL PALSY
IN SOCIAL GROUPS I–V

SOCIAL GROUP	CEREBRAL PALSY CASES	ENGLAND AND WALES LIVE BIRTHS 1949	SW. REGION LIVE BIRTHS 1949
	Per cent	Per cent	Per cent
I	3·5	3·5	4·4
II	20·9	12·5	15·9
III	49·6	57·3	53·9
IV	12·5	15·6	16·0
V	13·5	11·1	9·7

Possibly the significant factors from these figures are the higher incidence of cases in Social Groups II and V. It is purely conjectural whether the first figure can be explained by the fact that children are being born to parents of older age groups who may have progressed to Social Group II. The higher incidence in Social Group V might be related to the higher incidence of premature births which occurs in this social group. Obviously correlation between parity, age of mother, birth weight of child, and movement-defect type should be made, and this is not possible on these small numbers. Interesting figures could be compiled and correlations made if the numbers from many large centres could be added together. In this way an impression of mass aetiology could be obtained.

PLATE XVII

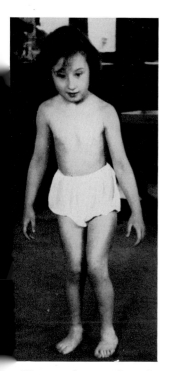

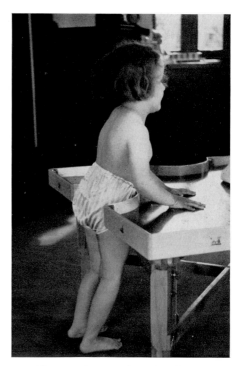

Fig. 30.—A case of ataxia
ith defective eye movements,
:neral flexion, and pes planus.

Fig. 31.—A case of ataxia with
hydrocephalus.

PLATE XVIII

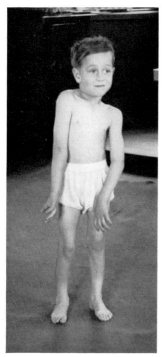

Fig. 32.—A case of athetosis showing effect of tonic neck reflex on eye movements.

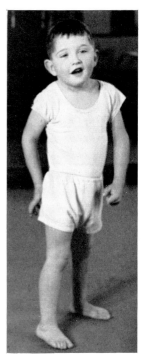

Fig. 33.—A child with athetosis who moves his head rather than his eyes.

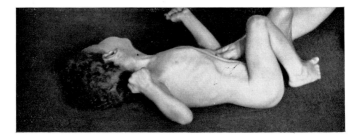

Fig. 34.—A case of athetosis with barrel chest and diminished respiratory flow due to abnormal posture.

CHAPTER XIII

VISUAL DEFECTS

FOLLOWING a detailed description of the seven distinct types of movement defect with very varied aetiology, it will be noted that in each category there are a number of cases showing visual abnormalities. These abnormalities include blindness, impaired vision, defective eye movements, and field of vision defects. These defects are, in most cases, neurological abnormalities directly related to the brain pathology.

The figures for eye defects are given below (*Table V*).

Table V.—VISUAL DEFECTS IN CASES OF CEREBRAL PALSY

MOVEMENT DEFECT	NO. OF CASES	BLIND	IMPAIRED SIGHT	MUSCULAR IMBALANCE	FIELD OF VISION DEFECT
Paraplegia	26	0	1	9	
Monoplegia	13		1	6	
Hemiplegia :					
congenital	69	2	8	11	5
acquired	28	0	4	5	5
Quadriplegia	75	2	19	40	3
Athetosis	33		1	17	
Ataxia	29		7	12	
Rigidity	28	5	5	10	

LITERATURE

The literature on eye defects in cerebral palsy is very limited, and most of the work has been done by Guibor in America, although Little noted the high incidence of strabismus in cerebral palsy in 1853. Guibor (1953 b) states that eye motor defects exist in 50 per cent of patients with infantile cerebral palsy, and observed that defective eye movements can accentuate defective bodily movements. Temple Fay (1954, personal communication) has noted the coexistence of a divergent squint with the persistence of a tonic neck reflex, relating both to his theory that in cerebral palsy there is a return to early embryological amphibian movements. Bobath (1955, personal communication) has demonstrated that some cerebral palsied children are unable to move the eyes independently of the head (*Fig.* 32), and has also observed the influence of persistent tonic neck reflexes on defective eye movements. Apart from these workers, there appears to have been little further study of the eye defects in cerebral palsy. In fact, Sorsby (1951) in *Systematic Ophthalmology* states that athetosis does not appear to affect eye movements—a very different finding from ours.

IMPAIRED VISION

As can be seen from the figures, cases of impaired vision occurred in this series in combination with all types of motor handicap. In quite a few cases the child was considered to be blind at birth, and only after a period of months or even years has it been possible to prove that some vision is present. In fact, occasionally, the vision has been found to be perfect in later childhood.

An inconstant observation in these cases of impaired vision has been evidence of a pale disk, suggestive of optic atrophy. This is a fairly common finding in cases of cerebral palsy and also in cases of mental deficiency (Norman, personal communication), even where there are no grounds for doubting the acuity of the vision. This finding may have little significance as the appearance of the disk in childhood is not clearly defined.

Observations on cerebral palsied children suggest that the impaired vision is cerebral and not ocular in origin. In many cases neither the parents nor the school staff can tell how much the child sees, and suddenly an apparently blind child appears to note the presence of something in the room, which could only have been ascertained visually. In some cases there may be damage to nerve-fibres leading from the retina to the external geniculate body or to the relay of the fibres to the occipital cortex. Apart, however, from the definite cases of field of vision defect in hemiplegia, there appears to be no clear evidence of partial field defects in cerebral plasy, and in the majority of cases the impaired vision is presumably cortical in nature. There is a defect in the functioning and co-ordination of the cortical centres concerned with vision, and the condition can more truly be called a visual agnosia or inattention. The child sees, but does not register his findings. There may be a cortical defect of visual imagery or the memory of visual imagery which prevents the child profiting by what he sees. In other cases there may be an inability to perceive the world in three dimensions, which will lead to marked visual confusion.

Some children who later appeared to have reasonably good vision showed either slow or no pupillary reaction to light in infancy, suggesting an extreme degree of visual disturbance allied to the auditory agnosia mentioned later.

There is a definite relationship between impaired vision and intelligence ; the 5 blind ' rigid ' children and the 2 blind quadriplegics were all ineducable. Some of these may be cases of bilateral hemiplegia of the parieto-occipital type. On the other hand, intelligent children with this visual handicap might be said to ' learn to see '. As they grow older and can move and crawl they learn to recognize visually distance, size, and texture and gradually sight improves. One such child was considered blind until 2 years of age, and then evidence of fairly good vision appeared. It may be that some of these cases of visual agnosia might benefit, in the early years, by definite training in the use of sight, and should be given ample opportunities to play and experiment with materials.

Many cerebral palsied children lack binocular vision. This may be caused by defective eye movements, mentioned later. In the case of non-brain injured children the lack of binocular vision due to a squint or uniocular damage does not appear to be a serious handicap. It is very likely not a serious disadvantage to brain injured children. On the other hand, some cerebral palsied children lack stereoscopic vision in the presence of both monocular or binocular vision. This may be due to occipital lobe damage and has some causal relationship with the child's inability to recognize pictures, shapes, and perspectives.

A cause of impaired vision in a premature cerebral palsied child might be retrolental fibroplasia. The combination of symmetrical spastic paraplegia or quadriplegia and retrolental fibroplasia is to be expected, and has been noted in 2 later cases, not in this series.   Ingram and Kerr (1954) have reported the combination of cerebral palsy and retrolental fibroplasia in 6 cases.

MUSCULAR IMBALANCE OF THE EYES

Another serious visual defect in cerebral palsy is a muscular imbalance of the eyes.   This defect was present with all types of movement defect in this series.   It is thought that the abnormal movements of the eyes were spastic, athetoid, or ataxic, according to the type of general movement defect in the child.   As suggested when describing the defect of movement in the limbs, the motor condition is an upset of total movement pattern, and not an abnormality of single muscles.   This is also true of the muscular imbalance of the eyes in cerebral palsy.   It is difficult to incriminate single muscles.   The whole nature of the eye movements is at fault.

Typically the spastic quadriplegics have a bilateral internal strabismus which is related to the adduction and scissors gait of the lower limbs ; but occasionally these cases show a divergent squint.   In an older child these deformities may have become fixed, and the muscles concerned permanently contracted in exactly the same manner in which a flexion contracture of the knees may occur.   In early childhood the spastic nature of the strabismus can be shown in that the eyes are capable, with relaxation and facilitation, of making a full range of movements.   As has been already noted, there is a high incidence of eye movement-defect in cases of paraplegia which followed a premature birth.

In athetoids the defect is one of conjugate deviation to one or other side.   The abnormality has some relationship to the persistence of the tonic neck reflex.   The eyes are typically deviated to the side of the strongest tonic neck reflex (*Fig.* 32).   In some of these cases there appears to be a slow nystagmus on frontal vision or on looking to the other side, and Guibor (1953 a) has suggested that this is due to the constant spasm in the eye muscles pulling the eyeball over to the preferred side.

Many of these athetoid or spastic children with deviating eye movements improve without any treatment as the control of the limbs improves. Quite a number of these children have been known to have a divergent or convergent squint as babies which has disappeared in later childhood. I have personally seen quite a number who show this improvement as the head control improves. In other children these defective eye movements lead to an alternating squint.

However, in some cases the spasmodic deviation becomes stronger and appears to be almost fixed. The child always looks sideways, and in doing so will move his head to see properly. In this way an ocular torticollis may develop, and the defective eye movements seriously upset the total movements of the whole body. The child walks with his head to one side, and with the abnormalities of arms and legs suggestive of persistent tonic neck reflexes. It appears obvious on first watching these children that they have seriously defective sight and are only able to see in certain directions. This observation may be quite inaccurate and, on examination, it is found that the child is capable of normal eye movements, and can see and measure distances showing hand–eye co-ordination with normal confrontation of the eyes. If this defective movement pattern is not corrected by training it may lead to a permanent strabismus, and also to defective vision. This is the eye picture which often characterizes cerebral palsied adults, and adds further to their abnormal appearance.

In some children of the ' ataxic ' group the child appears to have difficulty in holding the eyes in conjugate deviation, and as soon as the child moves its eyes to look sideways the eyeball springs back to the central position. These children have great difficulty in scanning a line of print when reading, and appear to have defective sight and pinhole vision. The same impression is given on walking, as the child appears unable to look to the side to see where he is going. On examination, it is found that these children are capable of normal lateral movements, but are unable to hold the eyes in that position for normal peripheral vision. It may be that there is a visual confusion on lateral vision and the child refuses to look sideways.

One particular child who showed this interesting difficulty also had many learning difficulties in the region of spatial perception, number sense, and a sense of body-image, all of which suggested parietal lobe damage. It may be that the disordered movement patterns of her eyes were also evidence of parietal lobe damage, and were in the nature of an apraxia.

Again, a further type of eye movement-defect is seen in some children who are capable of full eye movements, and yet find it easier to move their heads rather than their eyes. These children walk around shifting their head from side to side instead of making use of their eye movements, and the abnormality may occur in an intelligent child who is making good progress in other directions. It has been called " spasmus fixus " by Guibor (1953 a), and on carefully watching cerebral palsied children at play we find that the number showing this defect is greater than at first supposed (*Fig.* 33).

Thus it can be seen that defective eye movements can upset the movement pattern of the whole body, and treatment of the eye movement-defect must form part of the total programme in rehabilitation.

Another type of movement defect seen in cerebral palsy may be a nystagmus due to impaired vision. No case of nystagmus due to a midbrain or cerebellar lesion has been seen in this series, although cases have been reported.

In the eye movement-defects already described the suggestion is that the causal cerebral lesion is in the same region as the lesion causing the child's total movement defect, and not in the specific midbrain nuclei controlling eye movements. It is presumed that a lesion in the precentral cortical area or its tracts has led to generalized spasticity, and a lesion in the basal ganglia area to athetosis, both lesions involving eye movements. However, in a further type of eye movement-defect the lesion has been more definitely located in the area of the superior colliculus. As described in the chapter on athetosis (Chapter IX), some cases show a definite syndrome of an ataxic athetosis with high frequency deafness and defective upward movement of the eyes. The eyes in these children can move upwards reflexly, but they are unable to perform the movement voluntarily. The head control is poor, and the eyes tend to be prominent. The defect can be noted before the age of one year. Most of these cases give a history of neonatal jaundice and the cerebral lesion can be localized to a specific area in the midbrain, as shown by Wartenberg (1953).

FIELD OF VISION DEFECT

This visual defect is noted particularly in hemiplegic cases. It was noted in 5 out of the 69 congenital cases and 5 of the 27 acquired (postnatal) cases, although a few cases in both series were too young or too backward to be tested. Tizard (1953) noted that the defect is proportionally more frequent in acquired cases. The condition is an homonymous field of vision defect, and the lesion is in the optic radiation as it passes posteriorly in the depths of the parietal and temporal lobes to the occipital lobe, and has presumably been caused by a vascular lesion in the supply of the middle cerebral or posterior cerebral artery. In some cases, the visual field defect appears to be responsible for an internal strabismus.

Of the 5 congenital cases, 3 were educationally subnormal and the other 2 had a sensory loss and suffered from fits. Of the 5 acquired cases, 1 had superior intelligence.

There was evidence of a field of vision defect, either unilateral or bilateral, in a few of the quadriplegic cases. Presumably they could be considered bilateral hemiplegics. A field of vision defect may have been present in some ineducable cases, but it was impossible to test for this.

EYE-DOMINANCE

Lastly, the side of the dominant eye has a distinct bearing on the training of a cerebral palsied child.

In the normal population, 66 per cent (Pearce, 1953) to 69 per cent (Dunsdon, 1951) are right-eyed, and 34 per cent– 31 per cent left-eyed. In most normal people the dominant eye is on the same side as the dominant hand, but cross laterality occurs in between 37–46 per cent. When it occurs it is a mild disability upsetting the early attainment of the three Rs. It is felt that a normally intelligent child will readily overcome the handicap, but it may be an additional factor hampering the educational progress of a brain injured child.

The figures of eye-dominance are given below (*Table VI*). Many cases, particularly among the rigidities and the quadriplegias, could not be tested because of general backwardness. In other cases it was not always easy to be certain of the dominant hand due to the severe handicap.

Table VI.—Eye-dominance in Visual Defects in Cerebral Palsy

MOVEMENT DEFECT	NUMBER TESTED	RIGHT-EYED	LEFT-EYED	CROSS LATERALITY
Paraplegia	22	18	3	Per cent 9 (Numbers small)
Monoplegia	11	6	5	15 (Numbers small)
Right hemiplegia :				
congenital	39	12	17 ⎫	
acquired	11	6	5 ⎬	59
Left hemiplegia :			⎭	
congenital	27	24	3 (1 congenital cataract in right eye) ⎫⎬⎭	12
acquired	10	7	3 ⎭	
Quadriplegia	26	13	7	23
Athetosis	17	9	7	12 (1 left eye + ambidextrous)
Ataxia	22	13	9	19
Rigidity	Untestable			

In cases of congenital right hemiplegia there is a much higher incidence of left-eyedness than we would normally expect, and in left hemiplegia a higher incidence of right-eyedness. These figures appear to suggest that in cases of damage to the naturally dominant hemisphere, the minor hemisphere takes over both eye and hand, and presumably speech, control. There is suggestive evidence in this small number of cases that in acquired cases of hemiplegia the change-over of eye-dominance does not occur so readily.

In athetosis there is, as already shown, a high incidence of left-handedness, and this is associated with left-eyedness in many cases, although in severe athetosis this may be difficult to test for. B. Bobath (1954) has suggested that the left-handedness is due to a stronger tonic neck reflex on the naturally dominant right side, making the child use his left hand.

If this suggestion is correct, it may account for the high incidence of left-eyedness.

The figures in other movement-defect groups are small, and appear to be of no particular significance.

SUMMARY

The figures for visual abnormalities in the various movement-pattern defects are given.

The occurrence of blindness or impaired vision is considered to be cortical in origin and of the nature of a visual agnosia.

The muscular imbalance of the eye was due to spasticity, athetosis, or ataxia involving the movements of the eye-muscles.

The eye movement-defect can upset the movement pattern of the whole body.

In certain cases of athetosis there is a specific defect of upward movement of the eyeballs.

A field of vision defect was noted in some hemiplegic cases.

The side of eye-dominance may have some importance in cerebral palsy. Cross laterality may be an additional handicap to education.

CHAPTER XIV

AUDITORY AND SPEECH DEFECTS

FURTHER serious handicaps from which these cerebral palsied children suffer are defects of hearing and speech.

The figures are given below (*Table VII*).

Table VII.—HEARING AND SPEECH DEFECTS IN CEREBRAL PALSY

TYPE	NUMBER	HEARING DEFECT	SPEECH DEFECT
Paraplegia	26	1 (unilateral congenital defect)	3 (1 cleft palate)
Monoplegia	13	o	4
Hemiplegia :			
congenital	69	o	15
acquired	28	4	7
Quadriplegia	75	5	38
Athetosis	33	12	30
Ataxia	29	o	5
Rigidity	28	? mental defect	28

LITERATURE ON HEARING DEFECTS

Again the literature on this subject is very brief. The first published observation on deafness in cerebral palsied children was made by Phelps (1941). Since then separate groups of workers have noted the incidence of deafness (Coquet, 1944 ; Lande, 1948 ; Evans and Polani, 1950 ; Asher and Schonell, 1950). Perlstein (1950) particularly noted the evidence of high-frequency deafness in certain types of athetoids. More recently, Dunsdon (1951) in a small survey of cerebral palsied children attending a special school found a 10 per cent hearing loss in 60 per cent of the children. This high figure has not been found by other workers, and American workers have obtained figures of deafness in cerebral palsy in the region of 8 per cent (Beach, 1953, and Ziering, 1954). In his book *Auditory Disorders in Children* Myklebust (1954), very briefly, suggests that in cerebral palsy we may be dealing with a type of cortical deafness or auditory agnosia. This idea has been discussed slightly more fully by DiCarlo and Amster (1955). Lastly, Strauss and Lehtinen (1947) in their study of brain injured children have made interesting observations on the child's difficulty in synthesis and analysing sounds, leading to difficulties in reading.

Dublin (1951) reported pathological changes in the cochlear nuclei in some cases following neonatal jaundice, and Gerrard (1952 b) went further into an investigation of the possible pathology.

DISCUSSION

In giving the figures in cases of cerebral palsy the expression ' hearing defect ' is used rather than ' deafness ', because before making a diagnosis of deafness in these children it is important to analyse what we mean by the term ' deafness '. The condition is not one of peripheral or middle-ear deafness except in rare cases. It is also not a condition of nerve or inner-ear deafness. This condition more frequently occurs as the result of a congenital defect, or following treatment of tuberculous meningitis by streptomycin. The common hearing defects in cerebral palsy are of two distinct types, a high-frequency deafness and an auditory agnosia.

The cases of high-frequency deafness seem to occur more often in a definite type of athetosis—the typical ataxic athetoid— frequently associated with defective upward movements of the eyes. Here the lesion is in the cochlear nucleus. The hearing loss may be only partial and is rarely, if ever, complete. In many cases the deafness takes the form of a high-frequency loss. The child may have no prolonged delay in speech development but the speech is defective in the high-frequency tones of ' s ', ' sh ', and ' ch '. Some of these cases may be difficult to detect, particularly in the presence of a dysarthria due to athetosis. One girl spoke to me in simple sentences before she was 3 years old, and it was not until she was 10 years of age that it was found that she had a marked high-frequency loss and must be missing a considerable amount of the conversation around her. Another 5-year-old boy had a small vocabulary and only understood simple commands. He was thought at first to be either mentally backward or aphasic. He would shout and talk to other children and his partial deafness, which had seriously handicapped his language development, was only discovered when specifically tested for.

Other athetoid children are more severely deaf and develop no speech. In these cases, although the hearing loss is severe, it is never complete, and the child will suddenly turn to a sound —even quite a soft noise—if there are low tones in its composition. In this way it is very difficult to detect or get accurate figures of hearing loss. The majority of cases appear to follow neonatal jaundice. From the evidence of the small number in this series it would seem desirable that all cases of neonatal jaundice of every movement-defect type should be followed up to detect any hearing loss as early as possible.

In some cases it appears likely that the defective hearing is due to a cortical or subcortical lesion. The condition would be more correctly described as an auditory agnosia. The child can hear, but sounds mean nothing to him and he lives in a world in which he is ignoring all auditory stimuli. For neurological reasons which we do not fully understand, the child is cutting out the world of sound. There are a few cerebral palsied children of this type and in our series most have been athetoid. It has been suggested by Myklebust (1954) that the majority of cerebral palsied children with a hearing defect have this type of disturbance. It is presumably this type of defect which has accounted for the high proportion of cases of deafness in previous surveys. Unless, however, a satisfactory audiogram is obtained from every cerebral palsied child the exact figures of hearing loss due to cochlear nucleus damage, or to a cortical lesion, cannot be estimated. This full investigation has not yet been possible.

It has been shown by Strauss and Lehtinen (1947) that some cerebral palsied children have specific difficulties in synthesizing sounds and breaking down words into their components. This difficulty may increase some children's inattention to auditory stimuli.

An important factor comes out of this theory. If the defect in these children is one of auditory agnosia, the condition may be treatable. The child can be taught to hear and listen by prolonged periods of approach through the avenue of auditory experience only.   In the past ' cures ' of deafness have been reported by the Rudolf Steiner methods at their special schools. Their successes may have been in this type of case.   Miss Whetnall (1956) has shown that ordinary deaf children can be taught to use their residual patches of hearing if trained before the age of one year.   It may be that training these cerebral palsied children to use their capacity for hearing and discerning should start before 12 months of age.   DiCarlo and Amster (1955) have used the expression " perceptual atrophy ", and suggest that if the use of hearing is not encouraged the power may be lost altogether.

APHASIA

Literature.—The subject of aphasia in adults has been studied with precise classification and neurological localization by many workers, some of the original work being done by Freud in 1891.   Analysis of aphasic difficulties in children is considerably more difficult, particularly if they have never made use of the medium of speech.   The subject is discussed in detail by Myklebust (1954) and Kailin (1954).

Discussion.—In discussing aphasia in cerebral palsied children, the condition can possibly only be broken down into two types, sensory or receptive aphasia, and motor or expressive aphasia.

The condition of sensory aphasia, dating from birth, which is the ability to hear sounds but not translate them into meaning, is also called 'congenital auditory imperception'.   This condition may be distinguished from auditory agnosia, in which the child is hearing, but not even attending to simple noises.

A pure case of sensory aphasia has not been found in the series of cases among the congenitally brain injured children but has been found in 3 very premature children with no movement defect.   Quite a few cerebral palsied children are hearing but not understanding ; they are also not responding intelligently to their environment either visually or socially and therefore can be correctly placed as ineducable.

There appears to be evidence to suggest that the understanding of speech is located in the dominant hemisphere, with a subsidiary centre in the minor hemisphere (Goodlass and Quadfasal, 1954). It may be that in cerebral palsied children both centres are not equally damaged, and if the receptive speech centre of one hemisphere is damaged the other side can take over and truly become the dominant side. The figures on hand and eye dominance in the last chapter suggest this possibility. As these writers have suggested, at birth there are two potentially trainable language association systems differing slightly in readiness to learn.

On the other hand, sensory aphasia has apparently occurred in a few cases of hemiplegia and quadriplegia acquired after birth. On recovery from the cerebral catastrophe the child can hear but not understand. The ability appears to return gradually with training, but in a few cases, on intelligence testing, there is some evidence many years later of inability to understand.

In motor or expressive aphasia the child hears and understands, but is unable to speak due to a defect in the motor-speech area of the cortex. It is not due to a local movement defect of the organs of speech. Again, in our series, there was little evidence of this defect in the cerebral palsied cases which appeared to date from birth. The motor-speech area is considered to be in the frontal lobe of the dominant side, and again, it may be that if this area or the subcortical fibres leading to it from the temporal lobe are damaged at birth, the other hemisphere can take over speech control before the side of dominance has been fully established.

However, distinct cases of motor aphasia have been noted in cases of brain lesion after birth. It occurred in one child where the cerebral lesion took place at 8 months during an attack of pertussis and in another child who suffered from measles encephalomyelitis at 10 months. The condition was also noted in several of the acquired hemiplegic cases, but often there was additional evidence of sensory aphasia.

The first child, *Case* 10, attended a spastic school from the age of 3 years. The birth was normal, and his mother and family doctor considered that the child's difficulties dated from a severe attack of pertussis at 8 months. While at school it was observed that the child could hear and understand and had no difficulty in following gesture, and used it to make himself understood. He had no obvious perceptual difficulties and could understand pictures. At the age of 4½ years he was still unable to speak. This was not due to a local motor defect or emotional cause, but was presumably due to specific damage to the motor-speech area at a vulnerable time in the centre's development. He also had a left monoplegia.

These children can be taught to speak often quite successfully, presumably through training the other speech centre.

Thus, it is suggested that cases of pure sensory or motor aphasia may not occur, or if they do, very rarely, after brain damage at birth. They may occur after a cerebral catastrophe in later infancy.

SPEECH DEFECTS

In all surveys on cerebral palsy, the high incidence of speech defects is noted (Perlstein, 1953 ; Asher and Schonell, 1950 ; Pohl, 1950 ; Denhoff, 1955 ; McIntire, 1947) and therefore is only briefly mentioned here.

Apart from the cases due to high-frequency deafness, auditory agnosia, motor aphasia, mental deficiency, and a few cases of emotional origin, all the Bristol cases were due to a lack of motor control of the organs of speech. There was either spasticity, athetosis, or ataxia of the movements of the face, lips, tongue, palate, the organs of deglutition and respiration. Motor defects of speech were particularly in evidence in the athetoid group. In fact, in only 3 athetoid children could speech be considered normal.

For speech, the human race makes use of and adapts the muscles originally intended for breathing and feeding. It is not surprising that all cases of severe speech difficulties in later childhood gave a history of feeding difficulties in infancy : sucking, chewing, and swallowing had been difficult. A common movement defect in athetoid babies is that they extend their heads and protrude their tongues when feeding, thus pushing the teat or spoon out of the mouth. Many of the mothers of these children have resorted to pouring the food down their children's throats with no muscular effort on the part of the child himself. Thus, in later infancy, it is found that some intelligent children are unable to suck, let alone chew, and they have no control over the muscles of their tongue or lips. It is suggested that a speech therapist might help the mothers with the child's feeding movements in early infancy. In fact, the child should go through the normal movements of sucking, thumb-sucking, swallowing, chewing, babbling, preparatory to speech, in exactly the same way as the child should learn to roll over and crawl before walking.

This early tendency to protrude the tongue on stimulation of the lips or inside of the mouth may persist until later childhood, and in severe cases a spasm of the whole body may take place on attempting to manipulate the tongue. In other cases there may be a reflex spasmodic closure of the mouth on attempting to speak. A child of 5 or so years of age who appears intelligent may still have no speech, and may present the picture of motor aphasia or mental deficiency unless the condition is recognized. The child may even give up trying to speak. In other cases, on attempting to speak the child pushes back his head, extends his hips, and passes into a severe extensor spasm. Until he relaxes, he is unable to say what he wants to. The child may therefore give the impression of general slowness. This may not be due to a cortical dullness, but to a peripheral motor spasm. Any attempt to test these children's intelligence by timing responses with a stop-watch would be quite misleading.

In a similar way the lack of motor control may involve the respiratory muscles, and the child is unable to make a good voice due to an imbalance between the respiratory movements and the movements of the vocal cords (*Fig.* 34). Some of the athetoid children tend to speak on inspiration, resulting in a breathless talk. This respiratory inversion has been considered to be due to respiratory incoordination (Pohl, 1950) or to hypothalamic damage (Blumberg, 1955).

Possibly in some cases, the incoordination of the muscles of speech and respiration may be due to an apraxia, and the cerebral damage may be in the parietal lobe. Some of the few cases of speech defect in hemiplegia may fall into this category.

Other cerebral palsied children with either spastic hemiplegia, quadriplegia, athetosis, or ataxia have shown the condition of congenital suprabulbar palsy described by Worster-Drout (1953). They give a history of swallowing and chewing difficulties in infancy. The particular symptoms are defective movements of the palate leading to imperfect nasopalatal closure and a nasal speech, stiff incoordinated tongue movements, and persistence of dribbling. Some show poor lip and facial movements.

As many of these cerebral palsied children, particularly at adolescence, are facing severe problems due to awareness of their handicap, emotional speech difficulties can be expected. In this series, 2 adolescent hemiplegics, who were finding life adjustment difficult owing to fits, had a severe stammer.

Again, it must be recognized that in a fair proportion of cases, particularly among the quadriplegics and rigidities, the lack or immaturity of speech is due to a mental defect.

SUMMARY

It is suggested that two types of hearing defect are met with in cerebral palsied cases—a high-frequency deafness and an auditory agnosia.

Pure sensory or motor aphasia is rarely met with in congenital cerebral palsy. Cases may occur of aphasia of both types after a cerebral catastrophe in later infancy.

Speech defects in cerebral palsy are frequently due to a movement defect of the organ of speech and respiration, either spasticity, athetosis, ataxia, or apraxia.

CHAPTER XV

SENSORY DEFECTS

As mentioned previously, in the clinical condition of infantile cerebral palsy we are dealing with a wide variety of neurological diseases. It is, therefore, not surprising that apart from defects of movement and defects of the special senses such as sight and hearing there is also a loss of sensory appreciation. It was realized early in this survey that sensory discrimination should be specifically tested for wherever possible. However, in a fairly large number of cases the child was too young, too backward, or had not sufficient speech for adequate testing. The figures are therefore incomplete. (*Table VIII.*)

Table VIII.—Incidence of Sensory Defect in Cerebral Palsy

Movement Defect	Sensory Loss
Paraplegia	3
Monoplegia	0
Hemiplegia :	
congenital	23
acquired	13
Quadriplegia	5
Athetosis	0
Ataxia	3
Rigidity	?

LITERATURE

Phelps in 1941 was the first to mention that a sensory loss can occur in cerebral palsy and may materially affect the child's ability to use his limbs. His observations were made on hemiplegic patients. Stewart in 1948 noted a sensory loss in 16 out of 112 cases of hemiplegia in a mental deficiency institution. Many were too uncooperative to be tested. Tizard, Paine, and Crothers in 1954 carried out a detailed investigation of 106 cases of hemiplegia in America and found a sensory loss in 50 per cent with a slightly increased incidence in the acquired cases.

EXAMINATION

The sensory appreciations usually examined are those for pain, touch, temperature, vibration, two-point discrimination, sense of position, and stereognosis.

In this survey only an occasional case showed a partial loss of the sense of touch, pain, or temperature. A few of the older hemiplegic patients complained of a general dulling of sensation on the affected side. It was felt that this sensory loss was discriminative only and was presumably a cortical sensory defect. In a number of mentally defective patients there appeared to be a marked loss of a sense of pain which might be indicative of a gross cerebral pathology, possibly involving the thalamus.

Two-point discrimination is difficult to examine accurately in a young patient and can be considered as allied to stereognosis. It was therefore not specifically enumerated as a separate sensory defect.

A sense of position is particularly difficult to elucidate in a spastic or athetoid patient as the child has difficulties in imitating movement. It may be that a lack of appreciation of position is bound up with a lack of experience of normal movements. It is also related to a loss of a sense of body-image, as mentioned later. A lack of a sense of position in the toes was noted in some hemiplegic cases, but a good appreciation of position was found in quite a number of severely affected paraplegic, quadriplegic, and athetoid patients.

In this series the particular sensory defect that was tested for and enumerated was astereognosis. The child's appreciation of size, shape, weight, and texture was tested and his ability to synthesize these sensations into a correct guess of an unseen object placed in his hand. Synthesizing of varying sensations into a correct estimation of the whole object is a cortical function and in testing for stereognosis we are assessing the child's cortical sensory function. Although a loss of simple sensation is not to be expected, a defect in higher ability to analyse and synthesize may be encountered in brain injured children in whom the postcentral area has been damaged.

Quite a few intelligent children of 3 or 4 years of age will readily play a game of guessing what is put in their hands when their eyes are shut. In this way the presence of astereognosis can be readily detected, and the difference in the ability to guess an object in one hand and not the other may be very obvious. Definite figures of astereognosis could thus be obtained.

The findings are discussed under the separate headings of movement pattern defect.

Paraplegias.—In one child (*Case* 6) already mentioned, there was astereognosis in both hands. It had been noted that the child had a general awkwardness of the hands and tended to hold the fingers hyperextended. This might have been considered due to mild spasticity if the sensory loss had not been noted. In spite of the severe paraplegia, the sense of position in the toes was good.

In 2 cases of spinal palsy there was a loss of sense of position and vibration, an entirely different sensory loss from the true cerebral cases.

Monoplegias.—No case of sensory loss was detected in this group.

Hemiplegias.—It is in this group of cases that astereognosis in the affected hand is particularly in evidence and has been studied by several workers. Our figures of astereognosis detected by simple testing in a hemiplegic child yield similar figures. (*Table IX.*)

Table IX.—SENSORY DEFECTS IN HEMIPLEGIA

Type	Sensory Loss	No Sensory Loss	Untestable
Congenital hemiplegia	23	23	23
Acquired hemiplegia	13	6	7

Tizard (1953) noted a correlation between a sensory loss and a general undergrowth of the affected limb and also between a sensory loss and a visual field defect. All except one case of sensory loss in this series showed an under-growth of the limb. In some cases this was minimal, but in others it was very marked and the hand was noticeably smaller.

Fourteen cases, however, with no sensory loss showed a varying degree of undergrowth. The spasticity in these cases was very mild, mild, or severe.

In a few cases as described in the chapter on hemiplegia (Chapter VII) there was no sensory loss or undergrowth and very slight spasticity and yet the child refused to use the limb. It was presumed that there was a loss of body-image. In 2 cases a loss of body-image was present with a marked movement defect.

In some cases the undergrowth was out of proportion to the slight sensory loss and to the marked skill with which the child used the hand. Tizard (1953) commented on this type of case.

This group of cases with a severe sensory loss, loss of body-image, or an undergrowth of the limb corresponds with the three sub-divisions mentioned in Chapter VII.

All the cases with a visual field defect had astereognosis.

It has been suggested that because of this lack of sensory discrimination it is a waste of time to train the child to use his affected hand. Our findings do not agree with this statement. An attempt has been made to teach all the hemiplegic children to use their affected hand for such simple tasks as doing up buttons, tying laces, using a fork, opening doors, and as the assisting hand in craft work. There has been little evidence that a sensory loss is preventing a child from using his hand for these simple tasks.

Presumably an intelligent child learns to interpret the somewhat dulled sensation he receives from the limb and also learns to make use of his visual powers to assist his manual skills. Again, as previously mentioned, often where there is a severe sensory loss the spasticity is not so marked and vice versa. Thus, a hand with a sensory loss is often more useful and more cosmetic than one with a spastic motor defect. One child with a marked astereognosis and undergrowth of the limb was learning to play the piano and taking music examinations.

Our figures, although small, suggest that there was a higher incidence of sensory defect with acquired than with congenital hemiplegia. This finding was also noted by Tizard (1953) and may suggest a more gross pathology in the former group.

Quadriplegias.—In a large number of cases it was not possible to test for a sensory defect due to general backwardness. A definite astereognosis was detected in 5 cases, in 2 of which the condition was postnatal in origin and followed a cerebral catastrophe in infancy. All 5 were cases of asymmetrical quadriplegia. In at least 3 the condition might have been a bilateral hemiplegia. One particularly interesting, intelligent child (*Case* 25) with bilateral astereognosis is described in the chapter on quadriplegia (Chapter VIII).

In contrast to these few cases of sensory loss among asymmetrical quadriplegics and bilateral hemiplegics there was no evidence of astereognosis among the group of symmetrical quadriplegics following a premature birth. Their ability to recognize shapes quickly and accurately was in marked contrast to some of the hemiplegic cases, both unilateral and bilateral.

Athetosis.—No case of sensory loss was noted in this group. Even a child with a severe movement defect, who had never used his hands for everyday tasks, could immediately recognize a marble, a penny, or a hairclip put in his hand. This ability was all the more remarkable as the child had had little opportunity to use his hands for feeling or experimenting. In some way, by visual experience, he must have communicated an impression of feeling to his organs of sensation that could be translated into cortical memories. With these children there appeared to be no such thing as a virgin hand as suggested by Macdonald Critchley (1953 b). The ability of these athetoid children to appreciate and discriminate sensations indicates an intact postcentral area of the parietal lobe.

Ataxias.—In this group there were 3 cases of sensory defect. Two very interesting patients, *Cases* 37 and 38, have been discussed. They both showed the awkwardness and stiffness in the hands noted in the paraplegic child (*Case* 6). The condition had been thought to be due to a generalized spasticity until the astereognosis and lack of sense of position was noted. The older girl, *Case* 37, had realized her own difficulty and knew that she must use her eyes to help her hands. By her own perseverance she had learnt to play the piano and type and had passed through a Grammar School.

An astereognosis was also noted in an ataxic child where the aetiology appeared to have been neonatal jaundice. This child showed evidence of perceptual difficulties.

Rigidities.—There were presumably many gross defects of sensation in this group but they could not be elucidated.

DEFECT IN BODY-IMAGE

Apart from evidence of a loss of sensory discrimination in a surprising number of cerebral palsied patients, two other discriminative defects allied to a sensory loss have been noted. Quite a few cases appear to have a poor sense of body-image. This has been noted in their motor behaviour, as suggested in a few of the hemiplegic cases, and it may be noticeable in their drawings, as mentioned later.

It has been suggested by Albitreccia (personal communication, 1955) that the effortless, toneless, consonant-lacking speech in some spastic cases may be due to a defective body-image of the speech organs. Cerebral palsied children may use their jaw and respiratory organs for speech and make little use of their lips or tongue. Speech may be improved if slight pressure is placed on the lips or in the region of the vocal cords and the child is made conscious of the co-operation of these parts. Breathing may become more regular and co-ordinated if the child puts one hand on the therapist's abdominal muscles and one hand on his own to get a picture of respiratory movement. This incorporation of an idea of body-image into speech training may account for the success of training speech with movement and the value of curative eurhythmy where sounds are made to accompany movement.

There was no evidence of a loss of body-image in any of the athetoid children, but this defect may have been partially responsible for the incoordinated walk and bizarre movements in some ataxic children.

FINGER AGNOSIA OR GERSTMANN'S SYNDROME

Quite distinct from astereognosis, children with cerebral palsy may suffer from a finger agnosia—a condition in adults originally described by Gerstmann (1924). Blindfold, they are unable to state which finger has been touched. This loss, as mentioned later, is often bound up in adults with a difficulty in left-right discrimination, an acalculia, and an agraphia.

Only a beginning has been made in elucidating this factor in cerebral palsied children, but an attempt has been made to study it in children with learning difficulties. It has been observed that a child may suffer from astereognosis and yet show no evidence of finger agnosia. On the other hand, children with no astereognosis may show finger agnosia. In fact, several cases of finger agnosia have been in the premature quadriplegic group and it is this group of quadriplegics which does not show general sensory disturbance. Much more work must be done on this phenomenon, particularly with controls, but at present the tie-up between this syndrome and arithmetic difficulties is marked, and will be discussed later.

DISCUSSION

A sensory loss is a further neurological defect from which a cerebral palsied child may suffer. In the past, reports of sensory loss have only been made in the hemiplegic group, but in this survey it has been shown that a defect in sensory discrimination may be present in association with other movement defects and in fact may be responsible for defective movement. The sensory loss appears to be discriminative in type, and to be of the nature of a cortical defect. In Chapter XVII the particular learning difficulties which these children experience are discussed and the evidence suggests that with sensory and perceptual difficulties we are dealing with parietal lobe damage. The different types and degrees of defect may be an indication of different areas of parietal lobe damage.

SUMMARY

In 47 cases of cerebral palsy in the present series a sensory loss was detected.

Astereognosis was particularly in evidence in the hemiplegic group and there was a correlation between sensory loss, undergrowth of the limb, and visual field defect.

Astereognosis was also noted in some bilateral hemiplegic and asymmetrical quadriplegic cases, in 1 paraplegic and 3 ataxic cases. No case was detected among athetoids.

There was also evidence of a loss of body-image and a finger agnosia. Both might be considered as defects of sensory discrimination and could affect movement patterns and learning abilities.

The sensory defects were cortical in nature and suggestive of parietal lobe damage.

CHAPTER XVI

EPILEPTIFORM DISTURBANCES

AFTER a careful analysis of the child's total motor and sensory handicaps, the figures in previous chapters show that a high proportion of cases of cerebral palsy suffer from varying types of epileptiform disturbances. The figures given below (*Table X*) show the incidence of fits occurring after the neonatal period in the different motor defect categories.

Table X.—EPILEPTIFORM DISTURBANCES IN CASES OF CEREBRAL PALSY

TYPE	TOTAL No.	No. SUFFERING FROM EPILEPSY	PERCENTAGE INCIDENCE OF FITS
Paraplegia	26	5	19
Monoplegia	13	1	8 (Nos. small)
Hemiplegia :			
congenital	69	25	36 ⎫ 43 per cent
acquired	28	17	61 ⎭
Quadriplegia	75	37	49
Athetosis	32	6	22
Ataxia	29	8	27
Rigidity	29	16	55
Total No. of Cases	301	115	38

LITERATURE

The occurrence of fits among children with cerebral palsy has been noted by many workers, but few exact figures have been given. Sachs in 1926 found an incidence of 50 per cent and Yannet (1944) 68 per cent. In a selected group of children recommended for special school placement Dunsdon (1951) found an incidence of 14 per cent and a progressively higher incidence of fits in the low I.Q. ranges. She found a slightly higher incidence among athetoids (18 per cent) than among quadriplegics (17 per cent) or hemiplegics (16 per cent)—a widely differing finding from ours. Stewart (1948) in his series of hemiplegic cases found an occurrence of fits in 75 per cent. His cases, however, were all from mental deficiency institutions.

In reference to the nature of the epileptiform disturbances, Aird and Cohen (1950) showed that of the cases of spastic paresis having convulsions 55 per cent were grand mal in character, 23 per cent Jacksonian, and 22 per cent petit mal. Perlstein (1949 b) pointed out the frequent occurrence of petit mal attacks in athetosis due to basal ganglion damage.

PRESENT FINDINGS

The importance of epileptiform disturbances in infantile cerebral palsy can be noted from the fact that 115 out of the 301 cases had at one time or other suffered from a fit, an incidence of 38 per cent. In a few cases a single convulsion had occurred at a period of stress—either with hyperpyrexia or under nervous tension—but in the majority of cases the convulsive attacks were sufficiently frequent to upset the life and management of the child. If various forms of behaviour disturbance (discussed later) are epileptiform in nature the true incidence is even higher. Again, many of the children in this series are young and only a minority have reached adolescence. There is a distinct possibility that a number of the children now free from fits will be subject to attacks when they face the stress of school-life, adolescence, or adulthood. In fact during the period of this survey 9 children previously free from fits have had their first attack—all during school-life. Thus, judging from the figures obtained from this survey the final incidence of fits in cerebral palsy is higher than 38 per cent.

Various types of epileptiform disturbances have been encountered—grand mal, Jacksonian, and petit mal—and will be discussed under the headings of the movement defect.

Paraplegia.—Convulsive attacks of a grand mal type occurred in a small number of cases, but were markedly absent in cases of hereditary paraplegia and in cases following a premature birth. The only case in the latter group appeared to have had additional birth trauma, superimposed upon the original condition of paraplegia of prematurity. The other cases of fits followed birth trauma with hydrocephalus (2 cases) and meningitis (2 cases).

Monoplegia.—Only one case in our series with monoplegia manifested epilepsy. He was a premature, educationally subnormal child, suffering from petit mal. He was noted to have frequent falls which caused injury and he was originally thought to be ataxic. An E.E.G. revealed a spike and wave type of disturbance. On treatment the incidence of falls, in which presumably consciousness was momentarily lost, became much less.

Hemiplegia.—In contrast to the findings of Stewart (1948), in this collection of 96 cases of infantile hemiplegia there was an incidence of fits in 43 per cent. Our series includes, however, milder and more intelligent cases. On the other hand, the figure of 43 per cent must be considered an underestimate as it is known that fits may occur for the first time at any age, often years after the original cerebral trauma. *Case* 13, who was known to me from $2\frac{1}{2}$ years of age, had his first fit at 9 years. The fits later became so incapacitating as to prevent employment, and he was successfully treated by parieto-occipital lobectomy. One adult suffering from congenital hemiplegia had her first fit at 17 years of age.

The fits may be of varying types. In some cases they were Jacksonian in type affecting only the hemiplegic limb. In severe attacks the normal limb was secondarily involved. In other cases the attacks were grand mal in nature, varying from twitching of the limbs or rolling the eyes to a fully developed attack.

In 9 cases the attacks were petit mal in character and in 8 cases both grand mal and petit mal occurred. The attacks of petit mal were often not noticed or remarked on by the parents unless specifically asked. In a backward child the fact that he occasionally went " off into a daze " was not considered abnormal. These frequent petit mal attacks interfered with the child's education and could be a factor in the low educational attainment. In a few cases the psychologist first noted the attack while testing intelligence. There was marked all-round improvement with the treatment.

A fourth type of epileptiform manifestation noted in cerebral palsied children and particularly in hemiplegic cases was a hyperexcitable uncontrolled behaviour with an inability to concentrate. In several cases in our series convulsive attacks were also present ; the suggestion is that this behaviour may be epileptiform in nature. A case is briefly described.

Case 65.—The second child, born after a forceps delivery, weighing 7 lb. 2 oz. at birth. There were no recorded neonatal symptoms. Convulsive attacks first commenced at 18 months of age and occurred every 2–3 months afterwards. He had a mild right hemiplegia with astereognosis, no visual field defect, and an I.Q. of 80. He was a rosy-faced, happy youngster who showed frequent bursts of uninhibited behaviour. For instance, at 11 years of age, he would run up and kiss anybody and suddenly commit irresponsible acts such as taking the brake off a lorry. The E.E.G. suggested involvement of the left hemisphere with prominent theta activity from both temporal lobes. This disturbed behaviour prevented the child leading a normal life at home and school, and there seemed a strong possibility of future delinquent behaviour.

As shown in our figures and suggested by Tizard (1953) there is a greater liability to epileptiform disturbance after an acquired than after a congenital hemiplegia, suggesting a more extensive cerebral disturbance.

Quadriplegia.—The figure for epileptiform disturbance in this group was again high, 49 per cent. The disturbance was grand mal in character in every case, but 2 showed evidence of petit mal in addition. Many of the more backward quadriplegic cases showed frequent spasms of twitching, nodding, and vacant spells. These occurred many times a day and responded badly to treatment.

Athetosis.—In contrast, the occurrence of fits among athetoids was much smaller. Two cases had one convulsion only during a pyrexial illness in infancy. Two others had grand mal attacks. The E.E.G. in these last 2 cases showed abnormal waves from the cortical areas, suggesting a more widespread involvement than that of the basal ganglia only. Two others showed petit mal attacks, which is in keeping with the basal ganglia lesion.

Ataxia.—In this group of incoordinated, often educationally subnormal children, fits occurred in 4 children where there was a definite history suggestive of birth trauma. Grand mal attacks also occurred in 3 of the hydrocephalic children and in one case where there was a family history of epilepsy. The figures are small and the group a mixed one clinically so that it is not possible to attach much importance to the percentage incidence.

Rigidity.—The high incidence of fits of all types in this group is an indication of the gross cerebral pathology and runs parallel with the finding of a high incidence of epilepsy in mental deficiency hospitals.

FAMILY HISTORY

Our figures for epileptiform disturbances following cerebral palsy suggest that we are dealing with a different condition to idiopathic or hereditary epilepsy.

Peterman (1954) found that 50 per cent of cases with idiopathic epilepsy gave a history of epilepsy in the family. In contrast, in these 115 cases of cerebral palsy with epilepsy, only 8 gave a history of disturbance in other members of the family, and out of the 186 cases of cerebral palsy not having epilepsy 6 gave a history of familial epilepsy. It was felt that among the epileptic patients the condition might have been genetically determined in 3 cases. One was an epileptic athetoid, with an epileptic father. Another was the quadriplegic child (*Case* 23) mentioned in Chapter VIII, and one was an ataxic child.

When a case of cerebral palsy has occurred in a family, usually both sides of the family have searched their family trees for any evidence of neurological abnormality. In normal families the incidence of abnormalities is neither known nor discussed in the family circle. Any attempt to obtain the incidence of epilepsy in controls is likely to be an under-estimate. Yet a school medical officer who questioned parents at routine medical inspections found an incidence of 12 family histories (of at least one case of epilepsy) in 165 children. Some of these 12 cases may suffer from cerebral palsy; but the evidence suggested by these comparative figures is that the epilepsy in cerebral palsy is not usually genetic in type.

MENTAL DETERIORATION

It has been suggested that intellectual deterioration may occur after frequent fits and there may be an increase in the brain pathology. In the history of a few cases of acquired hemiplegia and quadriplegia a fit, in a previously epileptic child, has precipitated the paralytic condition. Apart from these cases, in our series we have no evidence of deterioration of intelligence after many years of inadequately controlled epilepsy. The majority of these cases have been educationally subnormal from early childhood.

In adult life, however, the occurrence of fits may be a more serious bar to employability than the movement handicap itself. The lack of employment may cause an apparent deterioration of the whole personality.

ELECTRO-ENCEPHALOGRAPHICAL FINDINGS

Literature.—Two groups of workers, Perlstein, Gibbs, and Gibbs (1946), and Aird and Cohen (1950), have studied the electro-encephalographic findings in infantile cerebral palsy. Aird and Cohen have shown that 85 per cent of spastics and 60 per cent of athetoids give abnormal findings, but that there is a focal pathology in only 32 per cent of athetoids. From a follow-up of their cases they suggest that if the E.E.G. shows no evidence of epileptiform disturbance the chance of a fit occurring is only 1 in 8. They found no correlation between an abnormal E.E.G. finding and the intelligence quotient.

Present Findings.—In this survey 175 records have been obtained. The full significance of the findings has not yet been assessed and must be the subject for further research.

The E.E.G. has been particularly helpful in making a decision as to whether an abnormal feature in the child's behaviour is epileptiform or not. A severe spasm or sudden cry may suggest a fit which the E.E.G. will illuminate and in the cases where epilepsy is suggested by the E.E.G., anti-convulsant treatment has been of benefit. The occurrence of a normal E.E.G. picture or one showing no epileptiform disturbance has in nearly every case been a true indication that the child is not suffering from epilepsy. However, in quite a number of cases the E.E.G. has predicted the future possibility of fits and these have later occurred in 9 children. It has been suggested by Denhoff (1955) that in cases such as these anti-epileptic drugs might be given to prevent this very likely occurrence. This policy has not been followed.

In cases of hemiplegia the E.E.G. evidence of overflow of epileptiform disturbance into the non-affected hemisphere must be considered a serious phenomenon and grounds for energetic treatment.

In other cases E.E.G. records have shown a temporal lobe disturbance which has usually, but not always, correlated with abnormal behaviour in the child.

Again the E.E.G. findings in quite a number of cases of cerebral palsy of all movement defect types have shown unusually quiet records and the significance of these findings requires further study. Various records of cerebral instability also require elucidation.

Throughout the survey a normal E.E.G. has been considered a good sign. This type of record has occurred in cases of paraplegia, monoplegia, and quadriplegia, following pre-maturity, and in quite a number of athetoid cases. Yet by contrast, a few cases of rigidity and spastic quadriplegia with mental deficiency give a normal record. The figures are not yet sufficiently complete for a full statement.

SUMMARY

Fits have occurred in 38 per cent of the 301 cases. This may be an underestimate. The epileptiform disturbances have been of all types, Jacksonian, grand mal, petit mal, and behaviour.

There was a high incidence among hemiplegics, particularly in the acquired type, quadriplegics, and rigidities.

The incidence was less in athetoids and in those cases tended to be petit mal in type.

The epilepsy appeared to be due to the cerebral trauma and not genetically determined.

There was no evidence of mental deterioration due to epilepsy. The E.E.G. was found to be a useful investigation and an analysis of the findings requires further study.

CHAPTER XVII

ASSESSMENT OF EDUCABILITY

FOLLOWING this description of movement defects, visual hearing and speech defects, loss of sensory discrimination, and epileptiform manifestations in cerebral palsied children, we realize that in many cases we are dealing with a multiple-handicapped child. Yet, over and above these physical defects, there is a disintegration of the child's whole personality which is usually translated as mental backwardness. This disorientation may involve a general loss of intelligence, a behaviour upset, or particular difficulties in learning.

LITERATURE

Several surveys have been made to assess the intelligence levels of groups of cerebral palsied children and of the intelligence of particular movement defect groups. Doll, Phelps, and Melcher (1932) analysed the value of different test materials in assessing intelligence in cerebral palsied cases. In 1946 McIntire in a total of 143 cases obtained the following figures : gifted, 0 per cent ; superior intelligence, 7 per cent ; high average, 12 per cent ; average, 29 per cent ; low average, 13 per cent ; dull, 13 per cent ; borderline defective, 8 per cent ; feeble-minded, 18 per cent. In 1951 Dunsdon carried out a survey throughout the country on cerebral palsied children who had been recommended for special school placement. She found, in particular, a high incidence of backwardness in athetoids ; 36·5 per cent had an I.Q. below 55. Floyer (1955) obtained the figures of intelligence for the cerebral palsied children of Liverpool and her results were similar to those obtained by Asher and Schonell in Birmingham in 1950.

Much of the literature on behaviour disorders following cerebral trauma has been written by Bender (1949). She has studied the behaviour sequelæ of all types of cerebral disorders, birth trauma, asphyxia, and encephalitis. Preston (1945) has also noted the behaviour problem following birth asphyxia. Rosenfield and Bradley (1948) followed up cases of birth asphyxia and asphyxia in pertussis and noted, in particular, the later evidence of arithmetic difficulties.

On special learning difficulties in cerebral palsied children much of the work has been done by Strauss and Lehtinen (1947) whose book on the brain injured child covers much that is at present known on the subject. Dunsdon (1951), Floyer (1955), and Cruickshank and Bice (1955) have also made contributions to the study of these children's particular difficulties in analysing and synthesizing concrete and abstract ideas.

Hebb (1941) analysed the effect of brain damage on intelligence in adults and in infants and came to the conclusion that birth injury had a more devastating effect on general intelligence than injury in later life. He did not find the same incidence of localized defects such as aphasia after birth injury, but thought the brain damage had caused a more general disorientation of the child's whole intellect. " Early injury ", he suggests, " may have a less selective and more generalized effect than late injury."

ASSESSMENT OF INTELLIGENCE

The intelligence of all the children in this survey has been assessed by Mr. R. V. Saunders, chief psychologist to the Bristol Child Guidance Clinic.

As explained previously, the aim in this survey has not been to obtain a definite numerical I.Q. for these children, but to place the children in the groupings, ineducable, educationally subnormal, normal, and superior intelligence, and after a fair trial to place these children in the most suitable available school.

The intelligence assessment has thus not been made on a single examination, but has been estimated or re-assessed after a trial period at school. The policy followed in Bristol is to allow all walking children to go to ordinary school at 5 years of age and to assess them for special education only if it has been proved on trial that the child's intelligence is sufficiently

9

below the normal level to require special school placement. Also in the last two years all non-walking cerebral palsied children have been admitted to the spastic school at 3 years of age unless it is genuinely obvious that they are not above the imbecile level of intelligence. In this way every child has had a fair trial and has not been assessed on a single examination. Quite a few of these children have shown evidence of more intelligence than a single assessment would suggest.

The general figures of intelligence in the various movement handicap groups are given below (*Table XI*).

Table XI.—INTELLIGENCE LEVELS IN CASES OF CEREBRAL PALSY

MOVEMENT DEFECT	NO. TESTED	INEDUCABLE Per cent	EDUCATIONALLY SUB-NORMAL Per cent	NORMAL Per cent	SUPERIOR Per cent	NO. UNCERTAIN
Paraplegia	25	20	16	56	8	1
Hemiplegia	92	11	27	53	9	5
Monoplegia	13	8	23	46	23	0
Quadriplegia	67	50	24	24	2	8
Athetosis	27	19	15	63	3	5
Ataxia	28	7	21	69	3	1
Rigidity	28	97	3			1

From this table it can be seen that in our survey some types of movement-pattern upset appear to have less intellectual involvement than others, but in every group except the rigidities there are marked exceptions. The table shows the fallacy of considering, for example, that because a child is a severe spastic quadriplegic he is necessarily mentally backward. One severe spastic quadriplegic, for example, had an I.Q. of 140, whereas 23 per cent of the monoplegics were educationally sub-normal. As Gowers noted in 1888, there is no relationship between the severity of the movement handicap and the level of intelligence.

COMPARATIVE INTELLIGENCE IN RIGHT AND LEFT HEMIPLEGICS

Some particularly interesting observations were made in comparing the intelligence of right and left hemiplegics. The figures are given below (*Table XII*) and are also represented in a graph (*Fig. 35*).

Surprisingly the left hemiplegics, who presumably in the majority of cases have suffered damage to their non-dominant hemisphere, show a lower intelligence rating. Hughlings

Table XII.—PERCENTAGE INCIDENCE OF INTELLIGENCE QUOTIENT RATING

INTELLIGENCE QUOTIENT	RIGHT HEMIPLEGIA		LEFT HEMIPLEGIA	
	No.	Per cent	No.	Per cent
Under 50	1	2·1	7	15·6
50–69	9	19·2	12	26·7
70–89	13	27·6	9	20·0
90–109	15	31·9	12	26·7
110–129	6	12·8	4	8·8
130	3	6·4	1	2·2
Total	47	100	45	100
Uncertain	3		2	

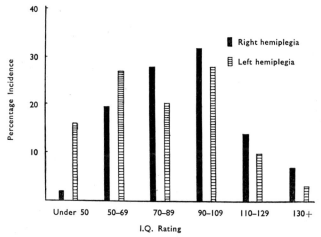

Fig. 35.—Showing the percentage incidence of intelligence rating in right and left hemiplegics.

Jackson (1892) made a slight reference to this finding and in a few of his cases of left hemiplegia considered that a lesion in the right posterior lobe was a factor in diminished intelligence. In his book Macdonald Critchley (1953b) gives definite functions to the minor non-dominant hemisphere, and suggests that the non-dominant hemisphere was the executive and the dominant hemisphere the storage of memory. A patient with damage to the dominant half of the brain forgets *what* to do, while the patient with a lesion of the non-dominant hemisphere forgets *how* to do it.

Possibly these findings in adults have some bearing on the difference in intelligence between left and right hemiplegics in children. The suggestion is that both hemispheres are of importance in the development of intelligence. The minor hemisphere is the seat of definite function, and damage will lead to a marked loss of intelligence.

BEHAVIOUR DISORDERS

After brain damage in infancy as suggested by both Preston (1945) and Bender (1949), there are frequently three severe behaviour disorders.

Lack of Concentration.—A brain injured child may be unable to keep his mind on one particular task for more than a few seconds and even then is readily distracted by what is going on around him. This is by no means true of all the cerebral palsied children. Some show quite marked powers of concentration and some will experiment and persevere with a particularly difficult task in a way unusual in normal children. This has been found true of the partially deaf ataxic athetoids and of athetoid children in general.

This lack of concentration may be due to a variety of factors. If the child is unable to focus or discern the objects around him, there is certain to be a lack of attention. If, on any sudden movement, the child goes off into a muscular spasm he may have lost the power of making an effort to concentrate. Because of severe educational difficulties which will be described later many apparently intelligent cerebral palsied children find the ordinary teaching methods too difficult for them and they cease to attend in class.

Our experience has been that if the education programme is kept within the child's ability to understand, this behaviour difficulty can be overcome. The child may be helped by short periods of individual teaching and when the three Rs have been mastered this lack of concentration is not such a serious problem in the classroom.

In a number of cases the lack of attention may be epileptiform in nature and due to constant abnormal stimuli from the damaged area. In some the E.E.G.s have shown abnormal foci in the temporal area and in some of these the attention span has improved with drug treatment. This type of brain-wave pattern may be found in all types of cerebral palsy but has been noted particularly in some hemiplegics and quadriplegics and one ataxic. In our series many of these children are also having true epileptiform attacks.

Hyperexcitability.—Coupled with this lack of concentration, there is in many cases a severe hyperexcitability. These children find difficulty in staying seated in an ordinary chair and in the classroom will jump up frequently to look out of the window. Allied to this hyperexcitable behaviour there is a more serious handicap of uninhibited behaviour. This was illustrated by the child (*Case* 65) already described. This behaviour is organic in origin and may be epileptiform in nature.

Perseveration.—This is a further characteristic of brain damaged children—" the persistent repetition or continuance of an activity once begun ". According to Strauss and Lehtinen (1947) frequently " after a good performance has been achieved, the organism, then confronted with a new task, continues to repeat the old performance ". For example, one of our paraplegic children aged 8 with a normal reading ability, had been playing with jig-saw puzzles, but when given an empty face and told to put the cardboard eyes, nose, and mouth on the face in the correct places, used the cardboard pieces purely as jig-saw pieces and tried to fit an eye in the curve of the hair as a jig-saw pattern. Frequent explanation that this was not a jig-saw did not deter her ; she could not stop the habit of doing jig-saws. In the same way a child may be unable to stop counting at the right number, or after writing a word correctly does it again and again, or continues to place beads in a board over and above the number asked for. This pattern of perseveration is a definite characteristic of brain damaged children and does not occur in normal or mentally defective children.

These three behaviour disorders suggest a total disorientation of the child's cerebration and an inability to organize separate and consecutive thought. It may be a factor in arithmetic difficulties, as suggested later. Apart from the excitability due to epileptiform disturbance from the temporal lobe, there appears to be no evidence to suggest which part of the brain is damaged.

LEARNING DIFFICULTIES

In addition to a lowering of general intelligence level and to the allied behaviour disorders there is also evidence in some of these children of perceptual and conceptual disorders which affect their ability to learn the three Rs. It is often translated as general mental backwardness, but may be due to specific brain damage.

In our Bristol Spastic School the teaching staff feel that the majority of these children with learning difficulties give the picture of a good brain damaged rather than that of a ' congenital idiot '. An attempt is made to elucidate the *clinical* nature of these particular perceptual difficulties.

Much of what we ourselves know in ordinary life has been learnt unconsciously. For example, a normal child of 18 months will look straight at a picture of a horse and say " horse " or " gee-gee ". He knows without learning that a picture in two dimensions can represent a three-dimensional horse. In some way that we do not yet understand these unconscious methods of learning have been denied to these cerebral palsied children and they have to learn in a painstaking, conscious manner things that a normal child appears to have ' been born knowing '.

" Perception ", according to Strauss and Lehtinen (1947), " is an activity of the mind intermediate between sensation and thought. It is the mental process which gives particular meaning and significance to a given sensation and therefore acts as a preliminary to thinking."

Most of the cerebral palsied children, excluding those genuinely mentally defective, outwardly behave and chatter in exactly the same way as ordinary children. They have good vocabularies, good verbal memories, their reasoning power is at the level of their chronological age, and teachers coming straight from an ordinary school class of the same age-group find the majority very similar to normal children in inquisitiveness, observation, and interests, provided always the child has had a social background similar to that of an ordinary child.

Yet sympathetic teachers and therapists dealing with these children note that many have some or all of the following learning abnormalities.

They may find difficulty in discerning up from down, right from left. They cannot distinguish round shapes from square. They are unable to recognize letters or pick out objects in pictures. They find it difficult to translate the three dimensions of ordinary vision into the two dimensions of pictures. They have not realized that a man standing up is a vertical figure in a picture and a man lying down is a horizontal figure. In the severest cases of impaired vision due to cerebral disorientation, they apparently cannot make sense of the three dimensions of ordinary life and in the worst cases they cannot recognize objects at all.

Some others have severe difficulties in the realm of number. In fact a lack of arithmetic sense has been shown to be a sequela of neonatal asphyxia by Rosenfield and Bradley (1948). These children may have no idea of number values. They may not be able to say that 4 is more than 3 and may be quite incapable of giving the correct number of articles on request. They find difficulty in visualizing the number as a group of pegs on a board, and cannot see which is a larger group and which is a smaller. This inability to deal with the simplest arithmetic can coexist with an ability to read and write up to the normal level for the child's age. It appears to be the one and only specific learning difficulty in some of these children and it may be that some children in ordinary school who are very bad at arithmetic, out of all proportion to their other learning abilities, have a slight brain damage. Some interesting work could be done on these lines.

In the executive field the brain damaged children often have more difficulties. They cannot copy simple shapes either on paper or with small sticks. They may even find up and down and simple slants or angles impossible to copy. The diamond shape in the Terman Merrill intelligence test which is normally performed by a 6–7-year-old may still be impossible to a much older brain damaged child. Writing thus becomes a great difficulty and some children who can read well are unable even to draw a simple cross. Oddly enough, some of these children can write simple words or stories if they wish to but are unable to copy. In copying, the words may be all jumbled up both vertically and horizontally.

Again, some of these children will do mirror writing, and one of our children occasionally would write upside down.

Their drawings may show disorientation. They will draw a man and put the legs on the other side of the page or draw a bus and put the wheels elsewhere. Proportions are often all wrong and too much is made of an unessential detail. In the milder cases the child may only appear to be a poor artist unless his efforts are carefully examined. In the severe cases the child appears incapable of making any organized shape with a pencil.

RELATED CLINICAL SIGNS

These odd perceptual difficulties appear to be partially related to some definite clinical signs which are described below.

Sensory Discrimination.—There appeared to be no marked relationship between astereognosis and the perceptual difficulties. Several hemiplegics with astereognosis and marked discriminative sensory loss showed no specific learning difficulties at school, and had kept level with their age-group in all subjects. On the other hand, several children who had no astereognosis and, in fact, were particularly smart at guessing objects put in their hands, showed many odd learning difficulties. This was particularly true of two symmetrical quadriplegics following a premature birth. In some cases, however, astereognosis and perceptual difficulties went together.

Cross-lateralism.—Cross-lateralism—one eye and alternate hand dominant—might account for some of the milder faults such as mirror writing, reversal of words and shapes, and a desire to write to the left and not to the right. Whether

PLATE XIX

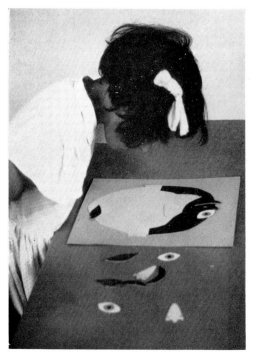

Fig. 36.—A case of ataxia, aged 8 years, showing the defect
in the idea of body-image.

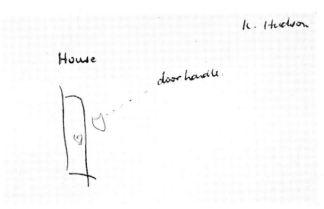

Fig. 37.—A drawing of a house by a child with spastic quadriplegia
following premature birth.

PLATE XX

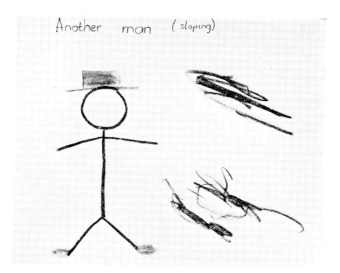

Fig. 38.—An attempt to copy a drawing of a man by a 6-year-old child with spastic quadriplegia following a premature birth. She has an I.Q. of 106 and is able to read.

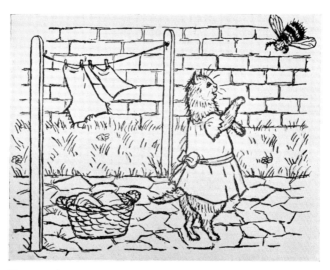

Fig. 39.—*Case* 69. Picture which 7½-year-old ataxic child, who could read, said was of a little girl riding a bicycle.

PLATE XXI

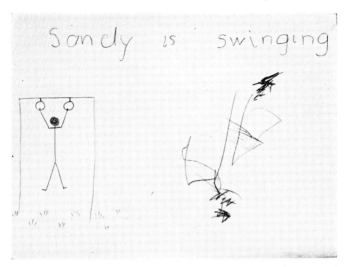

Fig. 40.—An attempt to copy the drawing on the left by an ataxic child of 8 years who is able to read. He had only reached this ability to draw after long practice.

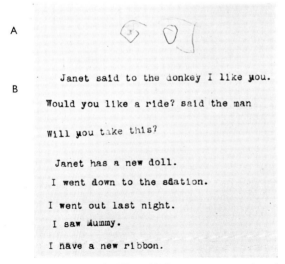

Fig. 41.—*Case* 67. **A**, The child's attempt to write the word " cat " ; **B**, Spontaneous typing, performed on the same day.

cross-lateralism is a serious handicap to an ordinary child is still in doubt and there seems evidence that even if it is an initial disadvantage an intelligent child soon overcomes it. It may be that to a brain damaged child cross-lateralism is a more serious disadvantage and augments the child's educational handicap. However, as the large majority of athetoids are left-handed and cross-lateralism is common among them, one would expect athetoids to suffer from perceptual disorders ; the majority of teachers of cerebral palsied children do not find these educational difficulties among their athetoid children.

Body-image.—Some of these children with particular drawing and movement difficulties appeared to have a lack of appreciation of body-image, as described by Macdonald Critchley (1953 b). Their inability to tell right from left, their attempts to draw a man, or to complete a test picture of a face suggested this handicap. Their speech and their walk often gave this impression. One intelligent hemiplegic boy drew one side of the body larger than the other and it would appear that the refusal to use the arm in some very mildly handicapped hemiplegics with no objective sensory loss may be due to a loss of body-image. The boy (*Case* 19) who suffered a right hemiplegia after an appendicectomy and always carried his arm away from and behind him, unless reminded, may have had the same defect. Possibly the defect in a sense of body-image gives a feeling of insecurity and accounts for some of the lack of concentration.

The loss of a sense of body-image is illustrated by a test devised by Albitreccia (personal communication, 1955). An ataxic child of normal intelligence, aged 8 years, was shown a face with eyes, nose, mouth, and eyebrows stuck on in the correct places. She was then given an exactly similar empty face and a selection of similar cardboard eyes, noses, mouths, and eyebrows and asked to put them in the correct places. Her attempt, shown in *Fig.* 36, with which she was quite satisfied, shows her total lack of power to execute or perceive a normal face. A spastic quadriplegia three years younger could do it perfectly and quickly.

Gerstmann's Syndrome and Finger Agnosia.—Some of the cerebral palsied children who have severe arithmetic difficulties show the symptoms of Gerstmann's syndrome. With a hand covered up they are unable to tell the examiner which finger is being touched. They appear to have a lack of body-schema of their individual fingers. Gerstmann (1924) found that this defect in adults was associated with a right–left disorientation, difficulties in calculation, and in the execution of letters. Some of the children in the Bristol Spastic School whom the teaching staff state to be unusually poor in number concept have shown this clinical sign quite definitely. In fact two children who have no astereognosis and few perceptual difficulties except for the poor arithmetic showed this sign particularly well, in marked contrast to younger cerebral palsied children who carried out the finger test without difficulty. More work is needed on these lines, particularly with the use of controls from a normal school. The overall suggestion is that in human philosophy the ability to count the ten fingers and ten toes is an essential basis on which to build a number concept, and when this power is upset by brain damage arithmetic difficulties result.

On the other hand, this last finding of a condition allied to Gerstmann's syndrome may be only a minor factor. Possibly a difficulty in consecutive thought and the presence of perseveration in the child's mental make-up prevent him forming a mental pattern of number.

These last abnormal findings—a loss of body-image and Gerstmann's syndrome—are thought to be due to parietal lobe damage, and to be comparable with the symptomatology of parietal lobe damage in adults (Macdonald Critchley, 1953 b). Several case histories are given below, illustrating different types of defect.

Case 66.—A symmetrical spastic quadriplegic child born after a premature birth, weighing 1 lb. 15 oz. Her I.Q. was 70–80 and she talked at 2 years of age. On first attendance at school at the age of 5 years the staff found that she could not understand pictures. In fact, they thought she preferred to look at them upside down. She had no idea of shape, jig-saw, or number.

At 7 years 10 months, after prolonged individual instruction she could read for me simple sentences such as : ' " What shall we play ", said Jill.' On testing, it was found that she knew and could point blindfold to her own nose, eyes, and mouth and those of the examiner.

When given a collection of pictures of pleasant and unpleasant faces and asked to sort them, her judgement was straightforward and perfect. Yet when asked to fit eyes, nose, and mouth into an empty face the result was no mouth and two noses. When asked to do a simple jig-saw of a man she made the legs come out of the arms. When shown pictures of men with missing parts she noted the unessential. For instance, with a man with an arm missing she immediately remarked that he had no hat.

She had no astereognosis, but showed a Gerstmann's syndrome on the left. In copying patterns with sticks, such as ⌐| |_ she was fairly competent, but showed some reversals |⁻ ⁻| . She could copy a few figures but had had practice. Her drawing of a house is shown (*Fig.* 37). She had little difficulty with rhythm or colour. Although her I.Q. was low, her perceptual difficulties came out in this test more than her low intelligence.

Case 67.—A symmetrical spastic quadriplegic child, weighing under 2 lb. at birth. At 3 years her I.Q. was said to be 112. At 6 years of age, she could read a number of simple words and had mastered the rudiments of arithmetic. She was left-eyed and left-handed and showed a tendency to reversals in copying patterns of sticks. She was critical of her efforts, and knew when she was making a mistake. Her sense of body-image was poor. Her main difficulty, however, was executive. Her left hand was good, and there was no motor handicap to delay drawing or writing, yet she was unable to copy the simplest shape, and her attempt to draw a man was a pure scribble (*Fig.* 38). She will need very specific training in copying shapes before writing is possible.

These last 2 cases are examples of the group of premature symmetrical quadriplegics described earlier. It is possible that they have a poor development of the parietal lobes. This group of cases responds well to special educational training.

Case 68.—A case of spastic paraplegia, following a normal birth. There was astereognosis in both hands, and she was right-eyed and right-handed. Her I.Q. was 75. At 8 years her reading ability was at least up to her age level, and yet she had no arithmetic sense. She had no loss of body-image ; her drawings of a man, and her detection of missing parts in drawings was good. In copying sticks, she showed frequent reversals. She was quite satisfied with |⁻| when asked to copy a square. She showed finger agnosia on the left hand which might not be outside the normal range for this ability. Throughout the testing she showed a marked tendency to perseveration. This particular child's difficulties were in arithmetic and in copying shapes.

The following case is described in greater detail.

Case 69.—A case of ataxia following neonatal jaundice and neonatal convulsions. He talked at 12 months, but did not walk until 4 years of age.

When 4 years old he appeared to be a dull ataxic child who took little notice of his surroundings. He showed an abnormality of posture, with flexed knees, flat feet, and general hypotonia. The physiotherapist said he behaved like a blind child. At 5½ years he was walking with poor control and still dribbled. The intelligence report was: "I.Q. 64. This result is an underestimate as the child was too distractable to test successfully. It was also doubtful how far he was able to see small drawings and objects, and this may have handicapped him to some extent. He gave only fantasy responses to the Pictive Vocabulary Cards, and held them sideways and upside down. The parts-of-body card he could see quite well, but his finger seldom pitched on the part named, although always very near. His speech is good, and he expresses himself well."

He was admitted to a spastic school at 5½ years, and it was soon noted that he was a child of some character with specific hearing difficulties. His verbal ability and reasoning were good, and he had a ' pretty wit '. His movement difficulty was one of ataxia, with general flexor spasticity. He still gave the impression of being partially sighted, and would turn the handle of a door by feel rather than by visual control, and would pick up objects from the floor without looking. Occasionally, he would nearly walk into a wall and correct himself at the last minute. He appeared confused in a room of furniture, and had difficulty in finding his way through it.

He could not be taught in an ordinary class because of his lack of attention. He was taught by short periods of individual tuition. In this way he learnt to read by the phonic method and grasped the idea of building up words phonetically. Later he could use the look–say method.

After a considerable period of pre-reading instruction in learning to recognize shapes, at 7½ years he could read simple words such as " fat ". By 9 years he could read, understand, remember, and enjoy simple stories in normal small print. However, he had to be continually reminded to look at the word. He had difficulty in focusing his attention at one point, and would make intelligent guesses. The scanning of a line of print presented problems to him.

However, coupled with the fact that he learned to read at an age not markedly above the normal, he continued to have difficulty in understanding pictures. At 9½ years he could just understand bold coloured pictures, but would often not notice an essential detail. When shown the picture in *Fig.* 39, he stated that it was a little girl riding a bicycle. This rather complicated black-and-white drawing was immediately understood by a symmetrical spastic quadriplegic boy of 3 years.

The patient also showed an executive difficulty in copying shapes (*Fig.* 40). His motor defect was not sufficient to account for his lack of skill. At 7½ years, when he could read simple words, he could not copy an X or an O. His attempt to write the word ' cat ' at 9 years is shown in *Fig.* 41, and this was after a considerable period of training. At the same time he could type and *Fig.* 41 shows his spontaneous typing done on the same day. He learnt the mechanism of a typewriter quickly.

He also had extreme difficulties with arithmetic. After prolonged training with modern educational devices, at 9½ years when asked : " You have six pennies ; I give you two pennies more—how many will you have ? " he answered " Five pence."

In ordinary school routine he had great difficulty in dressing himself, but this improved after practising on a life-sized doll.

This reasonably intelligent child, therefore, had the specific educational difficulties of being unable to recognize pictures, an inability to copy shapes, a poor number concept, and a difficulty in dressing himself.

The clinical picture is as follows :—

Eye reports : At 3½ years " slight pallor left disc, pupils active and equal. Both eyes fix for light. Sight probably good." At 7 years, difficulty in focusing, cerebral in character, sight difficult to test. At 9 years, the orthoptist found that he had full eye movements, and had binocular vision. He had no stereoscopic vision. He had difficulty in holding his eyes with lateral gaze on either side, and the eyes tended to shoot back immediately to the central position. As far as it was possible to test, there was no field of vision defect.

There was no evidence of cranial nerve defects except that he dribbled until 8 years of age. The reflexes in arms and legs were normal. The plantar reflexes were extensor.

At 8 years he had bilateral astereognosis. Finger agnosia was present in both hands and he had difficulty with right–left discrimination.

This case is described at greater length because it illustrates the problem of analysing and pinpointing the child's learning difficulties. It is thought clinically that these could be due to damage in the occipital and parietal areas.

There was no evidence of a peripheral defect in vision ; in fact he could read quite small print. Yet making use of the sense of sight appeared to confuse or be unpleasant to him and he preferred to have his eyes shut. His difficulty in recognizing pictures and in finding his way around a room suggested a muddled concept of vision in three dimensions. Possibly his refusal to maintain lateral vision was due to the confusion it caused. His visual world was so disorganized that he tried to cut out the world of sight. It may be that this is a case of congenital visual apraxia due to damage in the occipital areas. The E.E.G. which showed very slow delta discharges from the occipital regions would support this.

His inability to draw even the simplest shapes was presumably due to further cortical or subcortical damage. This might be due to a defect in oculomotor memory. However, a previous child (*Case* 67) had the same difficulty in execution, without any visual or occipital lobe symptoms. We may be dealing with a parietal lobe defect in the nature of a motor apraxia.

This child's defective sense of body-image could partly be explained by the visual difficulties, but the disorder appeared to go deeper, as he had difficulty in dressing himself. Associated with the astereognosis and finger agnosia this may be evidence of a parietal lobe defect. His faulty attempts to move around may be partly due to a lack of a normal concept of himself in space, and suggest the picture of parietal lobe symptomatology shown in adults.

The child showed a true Gerstmann's syndrome, with agraphia, acalculia, lack of right–left discrimination, and finger agnosia. His lack of number concept may be bound up with an inability to recognize his fingers. On the other hand, a full appreciation of number is an advanced concept, and may need intact perceptual abilities. Possibly his lack of appreciation of space and of himself in space fundamentally upsets numerical understanding.

One may wonder whether this child is a mild case of parieto-occipital damage similar to the bilateral hemiplegia of low intelligence mentioned in Chapter VIII. For some reason we cannot yet explain he had missed the full movement defect and had avoided complete mental deficiency.

These 4 simple cases show the wide variety of learning difficulties that cerebral palsied children may exhibit. In some cases, recognition of shape is particularly difficult. In others, it is the execution of shape that presents the problem. Other children, with neither of these difficulties, may have supreme difficulties with numbers. In others, the predominant difficulty is a lack of body-image.

Some cerebral palsied children had mild difficulty in learning the three Rs, others severe difficulty, and some brain damaged children appeared to be floating in space, neither focusing, understanding, nor co-ordinating their activities. On the other hand, some children have none of these difficulties. One severe spastic quadriplegic boy of just under 3 years drew me a cat as nearly perfect as could be expected. He obviously had no perceptual difficulties. He grew up to be of superior intelligence giving an I.Q. of 145, although at 11 years he was still unable to walk.

DISCUSSION

Three factors appear to interfere with the education of the cerebral palsied child. They are a lowering of general intelligence, unusual behaviour disorders, and specific perceptual difficulties. As a general rule, these three factors occur in spastic or ataxic patients rather than athetoids. Many athetoid children have a normal intelligence, and present no particular problems in education apart from their movement handicap.

The suggestion is that all these factors are due to cortical damage, and this is borne out by the fact that many cases of perceptual difficulties have presented E.E.G.s with evidence of cortical damage. Other cases have shown a quiet type of record which might suggest cortical immaturity.

The pattern of defect in our children follows so closely that shown in the work of Macdonald Critchley (1953 b) on parietal lobe disease in adults, that there seems evidence that these particular perceptual difficulties—upset of body-image and Gerstmann's syndrome—are signs of parietal lobe damage in brain injured children. This would possibly correlate with the fact that these symptoms may or may not be present with spasticity (precentral area) and astereognosis (postcentral area).

Other types of spatial imperception may be due to occipital lobe damage.

The evidence is that the behaviour disorders are related to defect in the temporal lobe and this has again been borne out by E.E.G. findings.

The lowering of general intelligence is presumably related to the sum total of the cerebral damage affecting the child's entire relationship to his environment, but again many of these children give an impression of specific learning disability rather than a total cerebral disorientation.

There are, possibly, two approaches to the problem of learning difficulties—a clinical and a psychological. In this thesis an attempt has been made to show that the difficulties are related to definite evidence of brain damage. The psychological approach may tie up these findings with difficulties in learning the three Rs occasionally shown by children in normal school, and the problems some normal children have in analysing and synthesizing shapes and sounds. However, it is felt that in some cases these difficulties are constitutional in origin and not quite comparable with the more concrete problems of brain injured children.

It is hoped that within the next few years, special research will be done in Bristol on these perceptual difficulties. There is a need to analyse the problems further and devise methods to help the children. For later life, it is as important to treat these perceptual difficulties as to treat the movement defect. These difficulties should be noted as early as possible, certainly in the pre-reading stage, so that many of the learning problems may be overcome before serious school work begins. In this connexion the policy of admitting children to a spastic school at 3 years will be particularly helpful.

Useful research can be done in correlating the type of learning difficulty with the aetiology of the brain injury. To find out whether, in fact, premature symmetrical quadriplegics have one type of difficulty and asymmetrical quadriplegics another. In this way some ideas may be obtained on the underlying pathology and on localization of these functions in the brain.

SUMMARY

The figures of intelligence obtained in this survey in the various movement defects are given.

There are some interesting figures on comparative intelligence of left and right hemiplegics.

Various behaviour disorders are discussed. Some may be epileptiform in nature.

The various specific learning difficulties are discussed and their relationship to definite clinical signs.

BIBLIOGRAPHY

AGASSIZ, C. D. S., O'DONNELL, M. B., and COLLIS, E. (1949), *Lancet*, **2**, 1030.
AIRD, R. B., and COHEN, P. (1950), *J. Pediat.*, **37**, 448.
ALBITRECCIA, S. (1955). Personal communication.
— — and TOURNAY, A. (1954), *Rev. Neuropsychiat. infant.*, **2**, 11.
ALEXANDER, L. (1942), *Res. Publ. Ass. nerv. ment. Dis.*, **21**, 334.
ANDERSON, G. W. (1952), *J. Pediat.*, **40**, 340.
APLEY, J. (1953), *Arch. Dis. Childh.*, **28**, 423.
ASHER, P., and SCHONELL, F. E. (1950), *Ibid.*, **25**, 124.
BAKWIN, H., and WEINER, A. (1947), *J. Pediat.*, **30**, 64.
BALF, C. F. (1948), *Arch. Dis. Childh.*, **23**, 142.
BARNETT, H. J. M., and HYLAND, H. H. (1948), *Nerv. Child*, **7**, 36.
BEACH, M. N. (1953), quoted in *Cerebral Palsy* (ed. Cruickshank, W. M., and Raus, G. M.), 1955, 195. Syracuse : University Press.
BEEVOR, C. (1903), Croonian Lecture, *Brit. med. J.*, 1909, **1**, 881.
BELL, J., and CARMICHAEL, E. A. (1939), " On Hereditary Ataxia and Spastic Paraplegia ", *Treasury of Human Inheritance* (Vol. 4, Pt. 3). London : Cambridge University Press.
BELNAP, W. D., MCKHANN, C. F., and BECK, C. S. (1950), *J. Pediat.*, **37**, 326.
BENDA, C. E. (1945), *Medicine, Baltimore*, **24**, 71.
BENDER, L. (1949), *Amer. J. Orthopsychiat.*, **19**, 404.
BENTON, A. L. (1955), *Child Develpm.*, **26**, 225.
BICKERSTAFF, E. R. (1950), *J. Neurol. Psychiat.*, **13**, 134.
BLUMBERG, M. L. (1955), *Amer. J. Dis. Child.*, **89**, 48.
BOBATH, B. (1954), *Physiotherapy, Lond.*, **40**, 259, 295, 326, 368.
— — (1955). Personal communication.
— — and BOBATH, K. (1950), *Brit. J. phys. Med.*, **13**, 121.
— — — — (1954), *Brit. orthop. J.*, **11**, 18.
BRAIN, SIR RUSSELL W. (1955), *Neurology*, Vol. 3. London : Butterworth.
— — (1956), *J. ment. Sci.*, **42**, 221.
BRASH, A. A. (1949), *Arch. Dis. Childh.*, **24**, 107.
BRINES, J. K., and LORD, E. (1939), *J. Pediat.*, **15**, 836.
BRISSAUD, E. (1895), quoted by Collier (1899).
BRITISH COUNCIL FOR WELFARE OF SPASTICS (1954). Addresses given at three-day Conference, London, Sept., 1954.
BRITISH MEDICAL JOURNAL (1951), Leading Article, **1**, 23.
BUCY, P. C. (1942), *J. Neuropath.*, **1**, 224.
BULL, J. W. D. (1949), *Brit. J. Radiol.*, **22**, 68.
BYERS, R. K. (1941), *Amer. J. Dis. Child.*, **61**, 915.
— — (1948), *Ibid.*, **75**, 433.
— — (1953), *Pediatrics, Springfield*, **11**, 174.
CAMPBELL, W. A. B., CHEESEMAN, E. A., and KILPATRICK, A. W. (1950), *Arch. Dis. Childh.*, **25**, 351.
CAPON, N. B. (1922), *J. Obstet. Gynæc. Brit. Emp.*, **29**, 572.
CARDELL, B. S., and LAURANCE, B. (1951), *Brit. med. J.*, **2**, 1558.
CARLSON, E. R. (1941), *Born that Way*. New York : McClelland.
CARMICHAEL, A. E. (1954), Lecture, British Postgraduate Medical Federation, London, Jan. 4.

CARPENTER, M. B. (1950), *Arch. Neurol. Psychiat.*, Chicago, **63**, 875.
— — and DRUCKEMILLER, W. H. (1953), *Ibid.*, **69**, 305.
CASS, M. T. (1951), *Speech Habilitation in Cerebral Palsy.* New York : Columbia University Press.
CAVANAGH, M. B., and THOMPSON, R. H. S. (1954), *Brit. med. Bull.*, **10**, 47.
CHILDE, A. E. (1953), *Amer. J. Roentgenol.*, **70**, 1.
CLIFFORD, S. H. (1947), *Amer. J. Dis. Child.*, **73**, 706.
COLE, W. C. C., KIMBALL, D. C., and DANIELS, L. E. (1939), *J. Amer. med. Ass.*, **113**, 2038.
COLLIER, J. (1899), *Brain*, **22**, 373.
— — (1924), *Ibid.*, **47**, 1.
COLLIS, E. (1947), *A Way of Life for the Handicapped Child.* London : Faber.
— — (1954), *Arch. Dis. Childh.*, **29**, 113.
COQUET, M. (1944), *Ann. pædiat.*, **163**, 83.
COURVILLE, C. B. (1950), *Bull. Los Angeles neurol. Soc.*, **75**, 129.
CRABTREE, N., and GERRARD, J. (1950), *J. Laryng.*, **64**, 482.
CRAIG, W. S. (1938), *Arch. Dis. Childh.*, **13**, 89.
— — (1950), *Ibid.*, **25**, 325.
CRITCHLEY, MACDONALD (1953a), *Brain*, **76**, 19.
— — (1953b), *Parietal Lobes.* London : Arnold.
CROME, L., KIRMAN, B. H., and MARRS, M. (1955), *Brain*, **78**, 514.
CROSLAND, J. (1951), *Arch. Dis. Childh.*, **26**, 92.
— — and MCKEITH, R. (1954), *Recent Advances in Pædiatrics* (ed. Gairdner, D.), 423. London : J. & A. Churchill.
CROTHERS, B. (1938), *Amer. J. publ. Hlth*, **28**, 3.
— — and WYATT, G. M. (1941), *Arch. Neurol. Psychiat.*, Chicago, **45**, 246.
CROWE, M. P. (1944), *Arch. Dis. Childh.*, **19**, 32.
CRUICKSHANK, W. M., and BICE, H. V. (1955), in *Cerebral Palsy* (ed. Cruickshank, W. M., and Raus, G. M.), 113. Syracuse : University Press.
CRUIKSHANK, J. N. (1930), *Causes of Neonatal Death.* Medical Research Council, No. 145. London : H.M.S.O.
DARKE, R. A. (1944), *J. Pediat.*, **24**, 148.
DENHOFF, E. (1955), in *Cerebral Palsy* (ed. Cruickshank, W. M., and Raus, G. M.), 21. Syracuse : University Press.
— — SMIRNOFF, V. N., and HOLDEN, R. H. (1951), *New Engl. J. Med.*, **245**, 728.
DENNY-BROWN, D., MEYER, J. S., and HORENSTEIN, S. (1952), *Brain*, **75**, 433.
DICARLO, L. M., and AMSTER, W. W. (1955), in *Cerebral Palsy* (ed. Cruickshank, W. M., and Raus, G. M.), 166. Syracuse : University Press.
DICK, A. P., and STEVENSON, C. J. (1953), *Lancet*, **1**, 921.
DOLL, E. A., PHELPS, W. M., and MELCHER, R. T. (1932), *Mental Deficiency due to Birth Injuries.* New York : The Macmillan Co.
DRILLIEN, C. M. (1948), *Arch. Dis. Childh.*, **23**, 69.
DUBLIN, W. B. (1949), *J. Neuropath.*, **8**, 119.
— — (1951), *Amer. J. clin. Path.*, **21**, 935.
DUNSDON, M. (1951), *The Educability of Cerebral Palsied Children.* London : Newnes.
EGEL, P. I. (1948), *Technique of Treatment for the Cerebral Palsied Child.* London : Kimpton.
ELVIDGE, A. R., and JACKSON, J. (1949), *Amer. J. Dis. Child.*, **78**, 635.
EVANS, E. S. (1946), *Proc. R. Soc. Med.*, **39**, 317.
EVANS, P. R. (1948a), *Ibid.*, **41**, 402.
— — (1948b), *Arch. Dis. Childh.*, **23**, 213.
— — and CHILDS, B. (1954), *Lancet*, **1**, 642.
— — and POLANI, P. E. (1950), *Quart. J. Med.*, **43**, 129.

FABER, H. K. (1947), *Amer. J. Dis. Child.*, **74**, 1.
FAY, TEMPLE (1953), *Amer. J. phys. Med.*, **32**, 338.
— — (1954a), *Ibid.*, **33**, 347.
— — (1954b), *J. int. Coll. Surg.*, **22**, 200.
— — (1954c). Personal communication.
FISCH, L. (1953), *Lancet*, **2**, 370.
FLOYER, E. B. (1955), *A Psychological Study of a City's Cerebral Palsied Children*. London : British Council for the Welfare of Spastics.
FORD, F. R. (1944), *Diseases of the Nervous System in Infancy and Childhood*. Springfield, Illinois : Thomas.
— — and SCHAFFER, A. J. (1927), *Arch. Neurol. Psychiat.*, Chicago, **18**, 323.
FREUD, S. (1891), *On Aphasia*, repub. London : Imago, 1951.
— — (1897), *Infantile Cerebral Palsy*, Spec. Path. Ther. (ed. Nothagel), **9**, 6. Vienna.
FRIEDMAN, J., GOLOMB, J., and ARONSON, L. (1950), *New York St. J. Med.*, **50**, 1749.
FULTON, J. F. (1945), *Physiology of the Nervous System*. London : Oxford University Press.
GARDNER, W. J. (1941), *Arch. Neurol. Psychiat.*, Chicago, **46**, 1035.
GARLAND, H. G., and ASTLEY, C. F. (1950), *J. Neurol. Psychiat.*, **13**, 130.
GELLNER, L. (1955), *Spec. Sch. J.*, **44**, 12.
GERRARD, J. (1952a), *Brain*, **75**, 526.
— — (1952b), *J. Laryng.*, **66**, 39.
GERSTMANN, J. (1924), *Wien. klin. Wschr.*, **37**, 1010.
— — (1940), *Arch. Neurol. Psychiat.*, Chicago, **44**, 398.
GESELL, A. L., and AMATRUDA, C. S. (1949), *Developmental Diagnosis*. London : Cassell.
GIRARD, P. M. (1937), *Home Treatment of Spastic Paralysis*. London : Lippincott.
GOODLASS, H., and QUADFASAL, R. A. (1954), *Brain*, **77**, 521.
GOODY, W., and McKISSOCK, W. (1951), *Lancet*, **1**, 481.
— — and REINHOLD, M. (1954), *Brain*, **77**, 416.
GORDON, F. H., and SCOTT-PEARSON, D. N. F. (1949), *A Survey of Cerebral Palsied Children in Northern Ireland*. Circulated privately.
GOWERS, W. R. (1888), *Lancet*, **1**, 709, 759.
GREENWOOD, W. O. (1924), *J. Obstet. Gynæc. Brit. Emp.*, **31**, 611.
GRIFFITHS, R. (1954), *The Abilities of Babies*. London : University of London Press.
GRISONI, A. COLLI (1954), *Courrier*, **4**, 55.
GRONTOFT, O. (1953), *Acta obstet. gynec. scand.*, **3**, 308.
GUIBOR, C. P. (1950), *Crippl. Child*, **30**, 4.
— — (1953a), *Amer. J. Ophthal.*, **36**, 1719.
— — (1953b), *Amer. J. phys. Med.*, **32**, 342.
HADRA, R. (1950), *Crippl. Child*, **28**, 18, 22.
— — (1955), in *Cerebral Palsy* (ed. Cruickshank, W. M., and Raus, G. M.), 294. Syracuse : University Press.
HAMMOND, W. F. (1881), *A Treatise on Diseases of the Nervous System*. London : H. K. Lewis.
HEBB, D. O. (1941), *Proc. Amer. phil. Soc.*, **85**, 275.
HÉCAEN, H., PENFIELD, W., BERTRAND, C., and MALMO, R. (1956), *Arch. Neurol. Psychiat.*, Chicago, **75**, 400.
HERLITZ, G., and BJORN, R. (1955), *Acta pædiat.*, Stockh., **44**, 146.
HERRON, R. Y., and EDWARDS, J. E. (1940), *Arch. Path.* (Lab. Med.), **30**, 1203.
HEYMAN, C. H. (1938), *J. Amer. med. Ass.*, **111**, 493.
HIPPOCRATES, *The Genuine Works of Hippocrates* (1849), Vol. **2**, 851. Trans. F. Adams. London : Sydenham Society.
HIPPS, H. F. (1948), *J. Bone Jt Surg.*, **30A**, 695.

HOLLAND, E. (1922), *Report on Causation of Fœtal Deaths.* M.O.H. Report 7. London : H.M.S.O.
— — (1922), *J. Obstet. Gynec.*, **29**, 549.
HOLORAN, I. M. (1952), *Brit. med. J.*, **1**, 214.
HUGHES, J. G. (1952), *J. Pediat.*, **40**, 606.
HUMPHREY, M. E., and ZANGWILL, O. Z. (1952), *J. Neurol. Psychiat.*, **15**, 184.
HUNTER, J. M. (1952), *Northw. Med., Seattle*, **51**, 403.
INGRAHAM, F. D., and MATSON, D. D. (1944), *J. Pediat.*, **24**, 1.
INGRAM, T. T. S. (1955a), *Arch. Dis. Childh.*, **30**, 85.
— — (1955b), *Ibid.*, **30**, 244.
— — and KERR, J. D. (1954), *Ibid.*, **29**, 282.
JACKSON, HUGHLINGS (1892), *Brit. med. J.*, **1**, 487.
— — (1931), *Selected Writings*, Vol. 2, 145. London : Hodder & Stoughton.
KAILIN, I. W. (1954), *Amer. J. Dis. Child.*, **87**, 752.
KEATS, S. (1954), *Brit. J. Phys. Med.*, **17**, 133.
— — (1955), *Amer. J. Dis. Child.*, **89**, 421.
KEITH, H. M., and NORVAL, M. A. (1950), *Pediatrics, Springfield*, **6**, 229.
KENNARD, M. A. (1940), *Arch. Neurol. Psychiat., Chicago*, **44**, 377.
KLAUS, C. (1954), *Brain*, **77**, 491.
KROHN, M. (1948), *Clinical Examination of the Nervous System.* London : H. K. Lewis.
KRYNAUW, R. A. (1950), *J. Neurol. Psychiat.*, **13**, 243.
LAMM, S. S., and KOVEN, L. J. (1954), *Pediatrics, Springfield*, **14**, 130.
LANDAU, W. M., and GILL, J. J. (1951), *Arch. Neurol. Psychiat., Chicago*, **66**, 346.
LANDE, L. (1948), *J. Pediat.*, **32**, 693.
LAURANCE, B. (1955), *Lancet*, **1**, 819.
LEHTINEN, L. E., and STRAUSS, A. (1944), *Amer. J. ment. Defic.*, **49**, 149.
LEVY, L. L., and ROSEMAN, E. (1954), *Amer. J. Dis. Child.*, **88**, 5.
LICHENSTEIN, B. W. (1940), *Arch. Neurol. Psychiat., Chicago*, **44**, 792.
LITTLE, W. T. (1853), *On Deformities.* London : Longmans.
— — (1862), *Trans. obstet. Soc. Lond.*, **3**, 293.
LITVAK, A. M., GIBEL, H., ROSENTHAL, S. E., and ROSENBLATT, P. (1948), *J. Pediat.*, **32**, 357.
LORD, E. E. (1946), *Children Handicapped by Cerebral Palsy.* New York : Commonwealth Fund.
McGOVERN, J., and YANNET, H. (1947), *Amer. J. Dis. Child.*, **74**, 121.
McGRAW, S. (1943), *The Neuro-muscular Maturation of the Human Infant.* New York : Columbia University Press.
McINTIRE, J. T. (1946), *Amer. J. ment. Defic.*, **50**, 491.
— — (1947), *J. educ. Res.*, **40**, 561.
McKISSOCK, W. (1951), *Proc. R. Soc. Med.*, **44**, 373.
— — (1953), *Ibid.*, **46**, 431.
McNUTT, S. (1885a), *Arch. Pediat.*, **2**, 20.
— — (1885b), *Amer. J. med. Sci.*, **89**, 58.
MAGOUN, H. W. (1951), *Quart. Rev. Pediat.*, **6**, 117.
— — and RHINES, R. (1947), *Spasticity.* Springfield, Illinois : Thomas.
MALAMUD, N. (1950), *J. Pediat.*, **37**, 610.
MARBURG, O. (1945), *J. Neuropath.*, **3**, 443.
MARSHALL, J. (1954), *Brain*, **77**, 290.
MEDICAL RESEARCH COUNCIL (1952), *Employment Problem of Disabled Youth in Glasgow*, Memo 28. London : H.M.S.O.
METTLER, F. A. (1955), *J. Neuropath.*, **14**, 115.
MEYER, E. (1950), *Crippl. Child*, **30**, 18.
— — and BYERS, R. K. (1951), *Amer. J. Dis. Child.*, **82**, 216.
MEYER, T. C., and ANGUS, J. (1956), *Arch. Dis. Childh.*, **31**, 212.

MILLER, E., and ROSENFIELD, G. B. (1952), *J. Pediat.*, **41**, 612.
MILLER, H. G., and STANTON, J. B. (1954), *Quart. J. Med.*, **23**, 1.
MINISTRY OF HEALTH (1949), *Neonatal Mortality and Morbidity*. Report on Public Health, No. 94. London : H.M.S.O.
MONCRIEFF, A. (1953), *Child Health and the State*. London : Oxford University Press.
MORLEY, M., COURT, D., and MILLER, H. (1955), *Brit. med. J.*, **2**, 463.
MUNRO, O. (1928), *Surg. Gynec. Obstet.*, **47**, 622.
MYKLEBUST, H. R. (1954), *Auditory Disorders in Children*. New York : Grune & Stratton.
NEILSEN, J. M. (1938), *Arch. Neurol. Psychiat.*, *Chicago*, **39**, 536.
NORMAN, R. M., (1933), *Mental Deficiency: Stoke Park Studies*, 153. London : Macmillan.
— — (1944), *Arch. Dis. Childh.*, **19**, 111.
— — (1947), *J. Neurol. Psychiat.*, **10**, 12.
— — (1953), *Proc. R. Soc. Med.*, **46**, 627.
OBHOLZER, A. (1951), *S. Afr. med. J.*, **25**, 741.
— — (1952), *Ibid.*, **26**, 653.
OSLER, W. (1889), *The Cerebral Palsies of Children*. London : Lewis.
PALMER, M. (1949), *Nerv. Child.*, **8**, 193.
— — (1952), *J. Pediat.*, **40**, 515.
PEARCE, R. A. H. (1953), *Arch. Dis. Childh.*, **28**, 247.
PENFIELD, W. (1954), *Brain*, **77**, 1.
— — and RASMUSSEN, T. (1950), *The Cerebral Cortex in Man*. New York : Macmillan.
— — and LIVINGSTONE, S. (1949), *Pediatrics, Springfield*, **4**, 157.
— — and ROBERTSON, J. S. M. (1943), *Arch. Neurol. Psychiat.*, *Chicago*, **50**, 405.
PERLSTEIN, M. A. (1949a), *J. Amer. med. Ass.*, **140**, 1232.
— — (1949b), *Nerv. Child.*, **8**, 128.
— — (1950), *Amer. J. Dis. Child.*, **79**, 605.
— — (1952), *J. Amer. med. Ass.*, **149**, 30.
— — (1953), *Pediatrics, Springfield*, **11**, 166.
— — GIBBS, E. L., and GIBBS, F. A. (1946), *Res. Publ. Ass. nerv. ment. Dis.*, **26**, 377.
— — and HOOD, P. N. (1955a), *Pediatrics, Springfield*, **15**, 676.
— — — — (1955b), *Ibid.*, **16**, 470.
PETERMAN, M. G. (1954), *J. Pediat.*, **44**, 624.
PHELPS, W. M. (1941), *J. Amer. med. Ass.*, **117**, 1621.
— — (1948), *Nerv. Child.*, **7**, 10.
— — (1949), *Ibid.*, **8**, 107.
POHL, J. F. M. (1950), *Cerebral Palsy*. Minnesota : Bruce.
POLANI, P. E., and McKEITH, R. (1954), *Guy's Hosp. Rep.*, **103**, 54.
POND, D. A., and BIDWELL, B. (1954), *Brit. med. J.*, **2**, 1520.
POSSON, D. P. (1949), *J. Pediat.*, **35**, 235.
PRESTON, M. I. (1945), *Ibid.*, **26**, 353.
PRICE, G. F. (1939), *J. nerv. ment. Dis.*, **90**, 51.
RIDDOCH, G., and BUZZARD, E. F. (1921), *Brain*, **44**, 464.
ROSENFIELD, G. B., and BRADLEY, C. (1948), *Pediatrics, Springfield*, **2**, 74.
RYDBERG, E. (1932), *Acta path. microbiol. scand.*, Suppl. 10.
SACHS, B. (1926), *Amer. J. med. Sci.*, **171**, 376.
SCHILDER, P. (1935), *The Image and Appearance of the Human Body*. Psyche Monographs No. 4. London : Routledge & Kegan Paul.
SCHREIBER, F. (1939), *J. Amer. med. Ass.*, **111**, 1263.
— — (1940), *J. Pediat.*, **16**, 297.
SCHWARTZ, G. A. (1952), *Arch. Neurol. Psychiat.*, **68**, 655.
SCHWARTZ, P. L. (1924), *Z. ges. Neurol. Psych.*, **90**, 263.
— — (1927), *Ergebn. inn. Med. Kinderheilk.*, **31**, 164.

SHERIDAN, M. D. (1948), *The Child's Hearing for Speech*. London : Methuen.

SHERRINGTON, C. S. (1906), *The Integrative Action of the Nervous System*. London : Constable.

SMALLWOOD, A. L. (1953), *Cerebral Palsy in Bristol*. M.D. Thesis, University of Liverpool.

SORSBY, A. (1951), (Ed.), *Systematic Ophthalmology*. London : Butterworth.

STEINDLER, A. A. (1935), *Mechanism of Normal and Pathological Locomotion*. London : Baillière, Tindall & Cox.

STEWART, R. M. (1942), *Proc. R. Soc. Med.*, **36**, 25.

— — (1948), *Edinb. med. J.*, **55**, 488.

STILLER, R. (1947), *Amer. J. Dis. Child.*, **73**, 651.

STRAUSS, A. A., and LEHTINEN, L. E. (1947), *Psychopathology and Education of the Brain Injured Child*. New York : Grune & Stratton.

— — and KEPHANT, N. C. (1955), *Ibid.* New York : Grune & Stratton.

— — and WERNER, H. (1939), *Amer. J. Psychiat.*, **95**, 1215.

STRUMPELL, A. (1884), *Jb. Kinderheilk.*, **22**, 173.

SYMONDS, C. (1955), *Brit. med. J.*, **1**, 1235.

TAYLOR, A. R. (1952), *Edinb. med. J.*, **59**, 70.

TAYLOR, J. (1905), *Paralysis and Other Diseases of the Nervous System in Childhood and Early Life*. London : J. & A. Churchill.

THOMSON, J. (1952), *Edinb. med. J.*, **59**, 45.

TIZARD, J. P. M. (1953), *Proc. R. Soc. Med.*, **46**, 637.

— — PAINE, R. S., and CROTHERS, B. (1954), *J. Amer. med. Ass.*, **155**, 628.

VAN EPPS, E. E. (1953), *Amer. J. Roentgenol.*, **70**, 47.

VESTERDAL, J., FOGHT-NIELSEN, K. E., and THOMSEN, G. (1953), *Acta pædiat.*, Stockh., **42**, 475.

VOGT, C., and VOGT, O. (1920), *J. Psychol. Neurol., Lpz.*, **25**, 627.

WALSHE, F. M. R. (1923), *Brain*, **46**, 1.

— — (1943), *Ibid.*, **66**, 104.

WARTENBERG, R. (1953), *Diagnostic Tests in Neurology*. Chicago : Year Book Publishers.

WEISZ, S. (1938), *J. nerv. ment. Dis.*, **88**, 151.

WERNER, H., and CARRISON, D. (1942), *J. educ. Psychol.*, **33**, 252.

WHETNALL, E. (1956), *Proc. R. Soc. Med.*, **49**, 455.

WILSON, S. KINNIER (1925), *Lancet*, **2**, 53, 169.

— — (1954), *Neurology*, Vol. 2, 891. London : Butterworth.

WORSTER-DROUT, C. (1953), *Speech*, **17**, 48.

WYLLIE, W. G. (1948), *Proc. R. Soc. Med.*, **41**, 459.

— — (1951), *Modern Trends in Neurology*. London : Butterworth.

YAKOVLEV, P. I. (1947), *Amer. J. ment. Defic.*, **51**, 56.

YANNET, H. (1944), *J. Pediat.*, **24**, 38.

YLPPO, A. (1922), *Klin. Wschr.*, **1**, 1241.

ZIERING, M. (1954), quoted in *Cerebral Palsy* (ed. Cruickshank, W. M., and Raus, G. M.), 1955, 192. Syracuse : University Press.

151

INDEX